Aromatherapy

Teacher Training

With Essential Oil

Rebecca Park Totilo

ISBN: 978-1-7343258-1-2
eBook ISBN: 978-1-7343258-2-9

HI, I AM REBECCA

I am so glad you have joined me on this aromatic journey of sharing essential oils with others!

Offering a short class in a relaxed atmosphere is a wonderful way to expose people to aromatherapy. Many of these same people often become customers, buying essential oils from you or taking another course.

The more contact you have with prospective customers, with an actual person behind the product, the more likely they will purchase from you. Presenting classes is a great way to market yourself and your goods with tangible benefits, whether your product is an educational workshop or an aromatherapy product. If you are asked to speak at a community center, those interested in learning more will return.

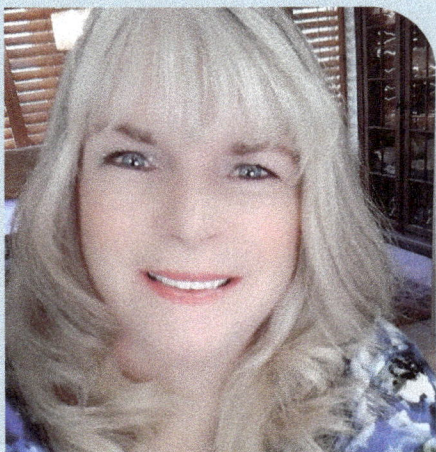

To make the class a memorable experience, be organized and ready! In this book, I am going to show you how to do that and much more!

CONTENTS

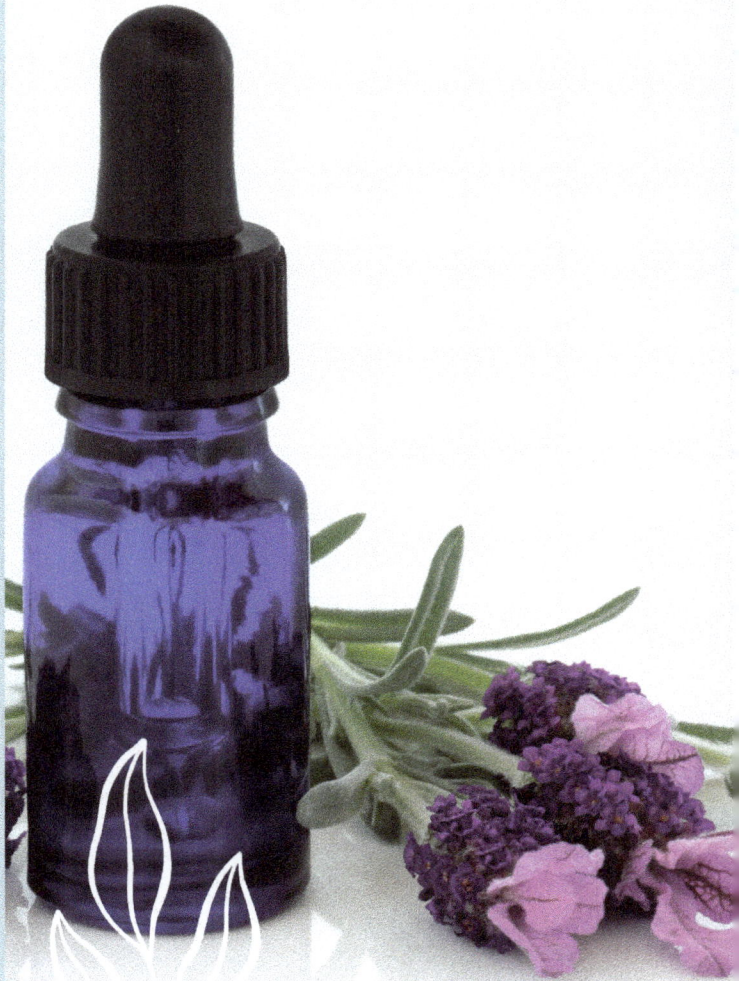

CHAPTER ONE —

THE
SCIENCE
OF TEACHING

Not everyone learns the same way. Some people learn by reading, some by listening, and others by doing. In this chapter, we are going to explore different ways that people learn.

LEARNING STYLES

First, let's start with some questions to get you thinking about your learning style.

- What helps you learn best?
- What helps you to remember? Do you need to see it, do it, or write it down?
- What has been hard for you to learn when it comes to aromatherapy?
- What was complicated about it, or why did you find it challenging? What do you think made it difficult for you?
- What was easy for you to learn and remember in your aromatherapy course? Why do you think it was easy?

There are three classes of learning styles, but some people overlap the various styles of learning.

AUDITORY LEARNER

An **auditory learner** is going to learn and remember things best by listening and by speaking. Students who are auditory learners greatly benefit from spoken lectures and talking through what they have just learned. These will be the students who raise their hands during class to repeat or summarize what was just taught. These students would rather attend a class when sick than relying on lecturer notes from their friends. Even if they study using written materials, they will grasp concepts better if they read notes aloud. You might recognize them from a class because they like asking questions, explaining concepts to classmates, or repeating what has been taught.

VISUAL LEARNER

Visual learners learn by seeing. They love graphs, charts, and pictures. Students who are visual learners love watching videos and watching others complete a task. Also known as spatial learning, people in this learning style prefers to use their eyes to grasp knowledge. They will focus more on written material and diagrams—they are often seen taking notes and doodling during a class. Visual students need time to process visual cues and do better with regular handouts and participation in writing examples on the board.

KINESTHETIC LEARNER

Kinesthetic learners learn best by doing. These are your students who seem to light up during the blending portion of your class. Once they put the information into practice, such as making an aromatherapy product, they understand and retain the information much better. Also known as tactile learners, they are the people who prefer to learn from experience or practical application. Such students are often quite active in class and will enjoy activities that require them to move from one point to another. A closer look at this type of learner indicates that they are active in outdoor activities and have an impressive class performance when fully engaged.

One other learning style we want to cover is **visual-auditory**

learners. These students will eagerly read the student handout and take copious amounts of notes during your presentation. Reading/writing learners understand concepts better when they are in the form of written words. Often overlapping visual learning, these learners will exhibit habits such as searching the internet constantly, making consistent diary entries, reading material posted on the internet, and looking up words in the dictionary.

You will have students in your classroom that have any of the above learning styles or a combination of all of them. This is why it is important to incorporate each of these learning styles into your course.

Knowing the learning style of an individual is of great benefit to both the teacher and the learner. This is especially true for students who are required to do a lot of self-study. Being differently gifted may seem like an inconvenience to someone who does not appreciate the uniqueness of human ability. Still, strength can be capitalized and minimized for someone aware of what they can do and how best to do it.

VISUAL-KINESTHETIC-AUDITORY CHART

The following chart can help you find ways to incorporate each learning style into your aromatherapy classes and workshops.

Visual	Kinesthetic	Auditory
Writes / Takes Notes in Class	Makes Blends in Class	Asks Questions About the Oils
Watches the Instructor Demonstrate	Passes Out Handouts	Listens to a Lecture
Draws a Chart	Smells a Perfume Strip	Says the Latin Name
Reads the Handout	Touches / Feels the Carrier Oil	Talks It Through the Classroom Distillation
Watches a YouTube Video on an Essential Oil	Volunteers to Pass Around Show–n–Tell	Practices Latin Names Pronunciation
Writes on a Whiteboard How to Calculate the Product Price	Helps Others Find a Recipe in a Book	Listens to a Podcast on Essential Oil Safety

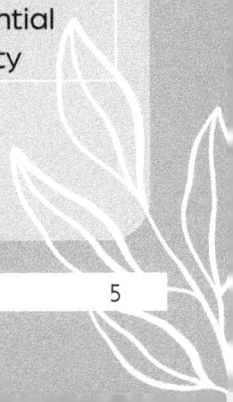

TEACHING STYLES

When presenting information to your students, your teaching can be considered active or receptive. In active teaching, you are creating what can be seen or heard. Receptive, or receiving, means to be taking things in. Let us look at the three main learning styles as it pertains to active and receptive instruction.

ACTIVE AND RECEPTIVE CHART

	Active	Receptive
Auditory Learner	Talking, anything that can be heard	Hearing and listening
Visual Learner	Creating anything that can be seen	Seeing, reading, looking, and watching
Kinesthetic Learner	Doing, being active with the body, expressing emotion	Feeling emotion, taste, receiving touch (massage), smelling

BLOOM'S TAXONOMY

Bloom's Taxonomy is a method for understanding effective teaching principles. When teaching using the principles of

Bloom's Taxonomy, your content will be organized into three key areas: knowledge-based, skill-based, and value change. You will want your class to include all three elements regardless of the length of the class.

Knowledge-Based Objectives — knowledge, principles, concepts, facts (Think Latin binomials, chemistry, botany, extraction methods).

Skill-Based Objectives — practical, learned skills (Think blending, formulating, consultations).

Effective-Based Objectives — effecting change in values and/or perceptions (Think love for plant-based healing, mind/body/olfaction connection).

When teaching a class, use all three objectives to have a well-rounded class that will grab and hold your students' attention and makes your class more memorable and powerful.

WHICH METHOD WILL YOU CHOOSE?

No two teachers will teach in the same way, just as no two students learn in the same way. A teacher's teaching style will be based on their educational philosophy, their classroom's demographic, what subject topic (or areas) they teach, and the school's mission statement. Reading through the list below, you can get a sense of the different teaching styles in traditional classrooms. You may feel led to adopt one of the principles as it is, a mix of several different principles, or you may develop your own teaching style that is 100% yours. There's no right or wrong answer here; it's whatever works best for you and your students.

The most important thing is to be yourself and find your own unique teaching style. You have unique abilities and gifts that no one else has—let them shine through and use them to make your classes as individual as you are.

Take a look at the list below and think about what kind of teaching style you have or want to develop.

TEACHER-CENTERED APPROACH

In the teacher-centered approach, the teacher is the authority figure, and the students are there to learn via lecture and direct instruction. The focus of this approach is mainly passing tests, and the teacher's goal is to pass information to students. There is one subcategory under this approach, and that is direct instruction. This approach allows you to use technology to teach.

DIRECT INSTRUCTION

Direct instruction is a traditional teaching model that includes teacher-led lectures and demonstrations. In direct instruction, the teacher's goal is to give students the information and knowledge they need to succeed.

There are three teaching models in this subcategory.

Formal Authority
Teachers are the authority figure and set the rules for the classroom. They are believed to have more knowledge than the students and hold a higher status than their students. Classroom

management is usually based on traditional methods involving teacher–designed rules and expectations.

Expert
Teachers guide and direct their students—they are the sole holders of knowledge within the classroom.

Personal Model
Teachers guide and direct their students—they are the sole holders of knowledge within the classroom.

Teachers lead by example. In this teaching method, the teacher leads by example and shows the student how to find information and understand it. This method allows the students to learn by watching and emulate what the teacher does exactly as the teacher demonstrates.

STUDENT-CENTERED APPROACH

Students can play an active role in determining how a subject is taught and learned. The teacher's job is to lead students and figure out the best way to teach the material.

According to some experts, the teacher is still the authority figure, but the student plays an active role in learning. The idea is that the teacher will advise and guide the students down a learning path. Assessment involves informal and formal methods—tests, group projects, portfolios, and class participation. The teacher continues to assess a student's learning even throughout the lesson. The students are learning the information the teacher is giving, and the teacher is learning how best to approach his students. There are two subcategories in this approach—inquiry-based learning and cooperative learning.

INQUIRY-BASED LEARNING

This teaching style focuses on letting the student explore and actively participate in learning. Rather than being a dictator, the teacher is a guide, giving the students advice and supporting their efforts. Students are expected to participate and play an active role in their learning. There are three models under this subcategory.

FACILITATOR

A facilitator teaching style facilitates the learning process. This teaching style is more hands-on, and the teacher's main job is to inspire students to explore and play an active role in their learning. This is a less formal teaching style.

Personal Model
This approach is similar to the direct instruction personal model subcategory. However, these personal models involve learning with the students while exploring and experimenting new ideas. In this model, students can learn that making mistakes is part of the learning process as they watch their teacher make mistakes. They will also see that people can learn from their mistakes.

Delegator
This teaching style puts most of the control into the student's

hands. The teacher provides the resources needed to learn, but it's ultimately up to the students to use the resources to understand what they need to know.

COOPERATIVE LEARNING

Cooperative learning is community-based learning. Students work together in groups to learn the material and complete any group assignments or projects. Most of the work in the classroom is group projects, and the students are responsible for their learning and development. This style's theory of teaching is that students learn best when interacting with their peers.

Facilitator

This model differs from the facilitator model under inquiry-based learning because it focuses more on group projects than individual work. The teacher still uses an open classroom, focusing on increasing a students' independence, hands-on learning, and exploration. However, instead of the student undergoing this learning process alone, they will share this experience with their classmates as a group.

Delegator

Like the inquiry-based delegator model, this model serves as a resource to students with a hands-off approach to learning. There is a greater focus on group projects than the inquiry-based learning delegator model. However, overall, the same key ideas are behind both models.

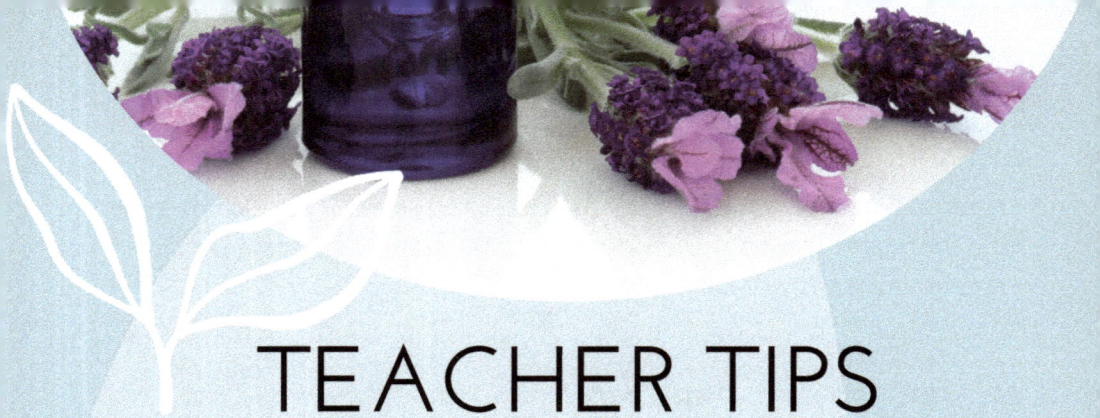

TEACHER TIPS

1

Know Your Audience

Who is your ideal audience for your class? What do they already know about your subject matter? What do they need to learn?

2

Managing Distractions

Ask for cell phones to be put on silent. Ask for questions to be saved until the end; hold a short Q&A session. Remember: You are in charge of your classroom.

3

"I Don't Know..."

Do not be afraid to admit when you don't know the answer to a question. "I am not sure about that; let me do some research and get back to you." Remember to get contact information and get back in touch with your student after researching the question!

4

Be An Inspiration

Ask yourself: how can I inspire this group of students? What does this group of students need from me? How can I best serve this group of students? Be a resource for your students!

5

Prepare

Take the time to plan your course and practice your presentation. Present your topic to a friend or family member. Did they understand your topic? What did they learn? Refine your presentation based on the feedback you get.

6

Go The Extra Mile

You can do this! Review your material and think about ways to improve your presentation.

7

Language

Cater your message to your audience. If you are talking to health professionals, feel free to use medical jargon if you understand what you are saying. If not, put things in layman's terms. Remember, for some students, you will be their first introduction into the world of aromatherapy, so keep information usable and straightforward.

8

Be Yourself

Let your personality shine through! You have something unique to offer the aromatherapy world and your students. Authenticity will create a stronger connection between you and your clients—they are more likely to like and trust you when they feel authentic with them.

9

Be a Resource

Supply students with information about where to buy essential oils, blending supplies, containers, etc. Always have another class planned before teaching—that way, you always have another experience to send students to. Recommend books, journals, websites, etc., for interested students to learn more about aromatherapy.

10

Have Faith in You

Always remember that you are a wealth of knowledge and have something great to offer the world. No one has what you have to offer—be you, share what you know, and be confident in your abilities.

CHAPTER ONE SUMMARY

As an aromatherapy teacher, your teaching style says something about you and your passion for essential oils. It is based on your values toward aromatherapy education and the philosophy you hold about essential oil education. Knowing how your aromatherapy students learn can also play a vital role in your teaching style. If you discover your teaching style early on in your career as an aromatherapist, both you and your students will be better off for it. You will understand your teaching preferences and how to reach your students' learning strengths in grasping the information.

Learning about and understanding the various teaching and learning styles can go a long way in helping you become a respected teacher in the aromatherapy industry. As you plan and prepare your course, you will see students be more engaged and develop a rapport with you when you keep these in mind.

Take time to demonstrate your knowledge of the various learning styles covered in this chapter. Prepare a short presentation or lecture (approximately 1-3 minutes long) on a topic such as "What is an Essential Oil" or "Safety Guidelines" using one of the teaching techniques covered above.

Remember to keep the different learning styles in mind as you prepare your brief lecture.

To begin:

1. Spend 5–10 minutes preparing your lecture. This can be on any subject related to essential oils; however, try to create one that will be your opening to a particular subject or topic for your workshop or class.

2. Choose an appropriate teaching method covered in this lesson to demonstrate. Use one in which you are comfortable with and feel is the best way to present your subject.

3. Choose a friend or partner to rehearse in front of several times (at least three times).

4. Ask your friend to critique you to help sharpen your skills and point out areas that need improving.

5. Before presenting in front of an entire class or group, consider which teaching style you will use.

6. Give your presentation. Be sure to make eye contact when speaking to your students.

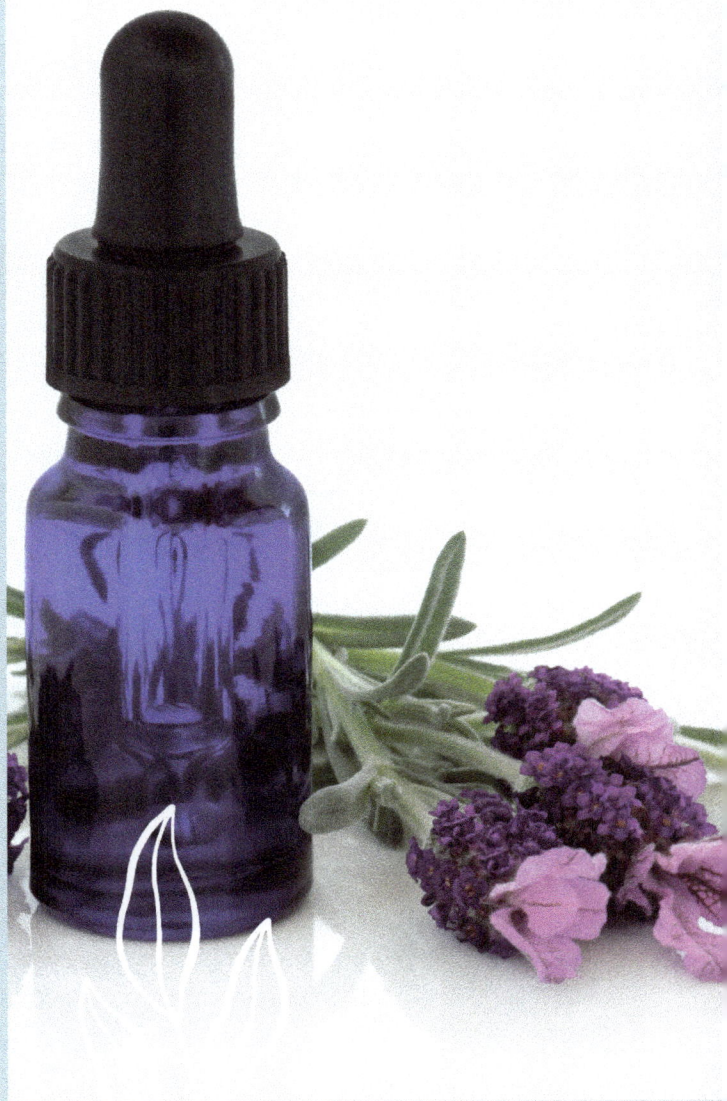

CHAPTER TWO ———

THE
CLASS

As an aromatherapist, you have a wealth of knowledge about aromatherapy and how to incorporate essential oils into your daily life. With that experience, your next step is to figure out how to share what you've learned with your students, some of whom may have little to no essential oil experience.

Begin by brainstorming about what you learned in your aromatherapy education. What topic in aromatherapy excites you? What do you feel qualified to teach about? What specific goal would you like to accomplish with your class? Is it going to be an introductory class for beginners or a more advanced class for people familiar with the topic? To answer these questions, let's examine some of the primary considerations you will want to explore in planning your course:

THEME

Having a theme will help you choose which essential oils to bring to your class and enables you to focus on the information you will share. For example, Rachel has planned a workshop called "Witchy Woman" to be held around Halloween with a topic that focuses on hormonal issues for women.

The following list is by no means an exhaustive list of the possible topics you can teach about. Use this list as a launching point for inspiration and see if you can develop other themes for your audience.

- Seasonal Threats and Allergy Support
- Cold and Flu Season
- Stress
- Anxiety
- Self-Care
- Green Cleaning with Essential Oils

- Essential Oils 101
- Sleep
- Essential Oil Spa Products
- Skin Care
- Hair Care
- Essential Oils for Pregnancy and Babies
- Essential Oils for Children
- Medicine Cabinet Makeover
- Mood Management
- Essential Oils for an Active Lifestyle
- Muscle Pain
- Travel Kit
- Immune Support
- How to Incorporate Essential Oils into Your Daily Life
- Essential Oil Safety
- Essential Oil Constituents
- How Essential Oils are Made
- History of Essential Oils
- Oils of the Bible
- Oils in the Antiquities
- Essential Oils of Egypt
- Aromatic First Aid
- Everyday Uses for Essential Oils
- Seasonal Essential Oil Uses
- Relaxing with Essential Oils
- Romantic Blends
- Holiday Blends
- Pain Management
- Essential Oils in the Classroom
- Aromatherapy and Learning Disabilities
- Disinfecting with Essential Oils
- Essential Oils as Antioxidants
- Cooking with Essential Oils
- Aromatherapy for Weight Loss
- Aromatherapy and End of Life
- Aromatherapy and Massage
- Aromatherapy and Reflexology
- Essential Oil Gifts and Crafts
- Essential Oils for Gardening
- Essential Oils for Pest Control
- Soap Making with Essential Oils
- Aromatherapy at the Office
- Aromatherapy and Animals
- Essential Oil Blending
- Aromatherapy and Beauty

- The Aromatherapy Home Spa
- Essential Oil Myths and Truths
- Essential Oils and DIY Diffuser Jewelry
- Essential Oils in the Medical Community
- Essential Oil Research
- Essential Oils and PTSD
- Natural Perfumes with Essential Oil

There are several products you can have your students make to practice their newly-acquired art of blending with essential oils. Your class theme will help you determine which products and essential oil blends to make in class. Below are a few examples of possible essential oil blends based on some of the main themes.

PRODUCTS TO MAKE

What kind of products will your students make? Below is a partial list of the types of products you can make in your class. Can you think of others?

- Bath Salts
- Salt Scrub
- Massage Oil
- Lip Balms
- Room Sprays / Linen Sprays
- Healing Balm or Salve
- Vapor Rub
- Roller Bottle Blend
- Hair Serum
- Scented Lotion
- Skincare Cream
- Liquid Soap
- Inhaler
- Diffuser Blend

Below are a few examples of possible essential oil blends based on some of the main themes.

- **Allergies:** inhalers, diffuser blends, room sprays

- **Digestion Issues:** roll-on, inhaler, diffuser blend
- **Colds and Flu:** inhaler, steam blend, chest rub, bath salt blend
- **Muscle Aches/Pain:** massage oil blend, body butter, salt scrub, bath salt blend
- **Everyday Living:** cleaning products, diffuser blends, body care products, linen sprays
- **First-Aid:** healing salves, hot and cold compress blends, antiseptic sprays, disinfectant creams
- **Immune Support:** diffuser blends, inhaler blends, hand sanitizer, liquid soap blend
- **Sleep Improvement:** room or linen spray blend, inhaler blend, bath salt blend, massage oil blend, lotion blend
- **Stress and Anxiety:** diffuser blends, inhaler blends, balms, roll-on
- **Household/Cleaning Products:** soft scrub, counter spray, glass cleaner, kitchen blends for sponges and cutting boards, all-purpose cleaner
- **Travel EO Kit:** hand sanitizer spray, inhaler blend, hotel room spray, roll-on blends for digestion or motion sickness

ESSENTIAL OILS

How many oils should you teach about? Which ones? When choosing essential oils to use in your presentation, be sure to select those that are easily accessible and affordable. Choose oils that you enjoy working with and never teach about an oil you do not have any experience with. Be sure to also take into account any safety considerations as well. The essential oils you choose to teach during your class are important. Consider each of the following questions below when selecting your oils for your class.

- Do you have experience with the oil? You should never teach about an oil that you have no practical experience with.
- How expensive are the oils you plan to teach about? You do not want to use expensive oils in your presentation that a student may love but cannot purchase due to cost. You will want to make sure your students can go out and buy the oils you teach about so that they will continue making blends on their aromatherapy journey.
- Are the oils you are teaching about readily available and accessible? Again, we want to make it easy for our students to purchase their oils to continue their aromatherapy journey. In many cases, if you are a wellness advocate or a distributor for a particular company, you will be using specific oils that your company carries and offer these for purchase at the end of your class.
- Do you have stories that you can share about the oils you have chosen? If you use oils, then you have a story to share. It is why we love them so much. Stories are a great way to connect your aromatherapy students with a particular oil. Even if you do not have a specific story about an oil, you can always share a friend's experience or a family member's story. Of course, do not forget to get permission before sharing about your husband's horrible toe fungus!
- Do you like the essential oil you have chosen? If you do not like an oil, don't teach about it. Your attitude toward the oil will come through in your teaching style.

- Always know the why behind the oils you have

chosen—you WILL get asked this by one of your aroma-therapy students.

- How many oils should you bring with you to class? The number of essential oils you bring with you to class will depend on the number of essential oils you will be teaching on and/or the products you will be making in class. Do not bring too many and overwhelm them!
- For a one-hour class, you may want to teach on three oils. For a two-hour class, you can cover six oils. For a three-hour class, you can usually cover nine to twelve oils. Depending on your timeframe, you can generally make one product in a one-hour class. In a two-hour class, you can make two blends, and in a three-hour class, you can make three blends. This is a simple guideline to follow and not a hard and fast rule. It can vary depending on how elaborate your products are.
- You will want to make sure you bring enough essential oil when creating products. For every five aromatherapy students, you will want to have at least one bottle of oil. So, for example, if you have twenty students, you will want to have four bottles of one particular oil, such as lavender, four bottles of peppermint essential oil, four bottles of orange, and so on.
- Make a list of all the essential oils you need to bring with you to class. Take into consideration the theme, the number of students, and if any products will be made.
- When blue-skying, make a list of all the essential oils you would like to teach about. Then, later down the road, you can use this list to choose from when planning your next class.

The number of essential oils you bring with you to class will

depend on the number of essential oils you will be teaching about and/or the products you will be making in class.

SUPPLIES

Your supply list will change based on the theme of your class and the product(s) you choose to make. Think through every aspect of the class and determine what supplies you will need to have on hand. Items that sometimes get overlooked include extension cords and other hardware. Teaching tools such as PowerPoint will require a computer, projector, and screen. Will you need a whiteboard during your lecture? Will Wi-Fi be available? Do you have any videos or audio you want to share with your students? Take everything you need for a class. Do not assume the venue will have what you need (always verify). If possible, set up a tote to be your mobile classroom to store all of your general supplies in it, so you are ready to go whenever you need it.

Make a list of all the items you will want to bring to your class. Consider what else you will need to have on hand for your class and add those items to your list. Gather these items ahead of time so you will be prepared:

- Essential Oils
- Essential oil books and Desk References
- GC/MS reports or profiles of the oils you are teaching about
- Carriers oils, Bath salts, etc.
- Bottles and Containers
- Computer and projector for presentation
- Plants, fruit, and resins; for example, cumin seeds, frankincense resins, citrus peels, or dried herbs or flowers
- Nebulizer or diffuser
- Paper Towels

- Coffee Beans (for clearing the palette)
- Glass bowls
- Tweezers
- Whiteboard or chalkboard
- Perfume Strips
- Sharpies
- White Labels
- Glass stir rods
- Bins to hold oils
- Snacks
- Gift bags
- Name Tags
- Door Prizes
- Brochures about your business or business cards

OUTLINE

Create an outline for the class you are planning. Use the outline to develop your content and keep your class on point. What main points do you need to make to help them understand the topic you are teaching? Make a long list, then choose which points you feel are the most relevant to your audience.

As a trained aromatherapist, you have had the opportunity to integrate a tremendous amount of information with hands-on experience. Now, as a teacher of aromatherapy, it will be vital for you to convey that information to your students and clients, who are just getting acquainted with essential oils.

See the section on Planning Your Class for more information about creating an outline.

HANDOUTS

Offer written materials for students to take home and refer to later on. You will want to provide a handout for each student with information about the course material you will be covering. Here are some other items you may want to include on your handouts:

- Short datasheets for the oils you are teaching – this can be as simple as a common name, Latin name, country of origin, plant part, extraction method, safety, and a few suggested uses for the oil. Basic, general safety information on using essential oils
- Blending dilution guidelines (rate chart)
- A few basic recipes
- A short, recommended book list (3–4 books appropriate for the level of student you are presenting to)
- A resource list of essential oil wholesalers, bottles, and carrier oils
- Your marketing materials (may be as simple as your contact information and a list of products/services you offer) Several websites and blogs for more information about essential oils (yours, NAHA, and a few others)

VENUES

There are many great places for hosting your short class or workshop—some will be free, and others may come with a fee. Choose a few places you would like to hold classes and find out what prices they charge and other details for renting their space. Having this information will help you in your decision-making process. Here are a few ideas for venues:

- Yacht clubs
- Hospice centers
- Massage chapter meetings
- Chiropractic offices
- Alternative educational schools (massage, chiropractor, esthetician, acupuncture)
- Community centers

- Local co-op or health food store
- Local spa staff day

- Health fairs
- Local libraries
- RV parks
- Recreational centers

- Hotel meeting rooms
- Restaurants (many have meeting rooms)
- Local government or Fire halls
- Salons
- Coffee shops

Of course, each area will be different, and you may have other ideas for where to hold classes. Be creative; keep in mind where you host your class can say as much about you and your business as the content you are teaching.

ICE BREAKERS

When the attendees arrive at your class, you want to make them feel at ease and relaxed. Greet each one and try to make a connection. After everyone has settled in at the beginning of your class, it's always fun to do an ice breaker to help students get to know each other while creating a sense of community with your students. Below is a list of icebreakers you can try:

- Which oil am I? Place name tag with oil name on the back of each person, and the person has to ask others questions to figure out which oil they are.
- Matching Pairs game (with oil and plant)
- Guess the scent (bottle of essential oil without label)
- What is your favorite scent?
- Who got you to come to the class today?
- Share your favorite aroma memory
- Share something new and good in your life
- Share your intention for taking this class

- Write with three things about yourself on a card. Place the card on the table, and each person chooses one and tries to figure out who it is.

At the end of the class, ask participants to share a favorite aroma memory. This will bring everyone together again, and everyone leaves in a thoughtful, memorable way versus everyone rushing out the door in a hectic way. Depending on the theme of your class, you may want to close in prayer or with music and a diffuser filled with relaxing fragrance. This will, of course, depend on the mood you want to create and the atmosphere you are working in.

PLANNING YOUR CLASS

Planning your class is one of the most important functions of being an aromatherapy teacher. How you plan and present your material will determine how memorable it is for your students and how much they learn. This, of course, will factor into having repeat students and referrals for future students. Creating your lesson plan is a crucial step in teaching aromatherapy classes. To be fully prepared, you have to know what you will teach and how you will teach it. Let's talk about your class's structure (which is the backbone) and how to develop your lesson plan.

The topics that can be taught surrounding aromatherapy are nearly endless. It is best to pick an idea that interests you because your interest in the subject will come through in your teaching. Also, remember that your topic needs to work with your target audience—it does not make much sense to teach a class on essential oils for kids to a group of high schoolers. Take the time to prepare for your class. This will help your class run more smoothly while boosting your confidence level in the early days of teaching.

CHOOSE YOUR TOPIC

Be specific about what you will teach. For example: If you say, "I want to teach about essential oils," this is too general. A topic too general can be too much information, leaving you and the student feeling overwhelmed. Instead, if you say, "I want to teach about Cleaning with Essential Oil in the Home," this is specific.

LEARN EVERYTHING ABOUT YOUR TOPIC

Here are a few questions to ask yourself. What are you going to teach about? What do you not know or understand about that topic? What information will you need to know to present this information to your class? You will want to learn all you can about a topic and have enough experience with the topic to share your expertise readily.

For example, if your topic was "Cleaning With Essential Oils," here are some things to consider:

- *Where can I find great cleaning recipes?
- *What ingredients can I safely mix together to clean with?
- *Why is cleaning with essential oil better than using regular household cleaners?
- *Where do I find containers for storing the essential oil products we make?

Have a specific plan for presenting your knowledge and experience in a way that will achieve your goal.

SET A GOAL FOR YOUR CLASS

What is the specific goal for the class? What message or action do you want your class members to take away once your class is over? Do you want them to purchase essential oils? Or sign up for another course? Your goal will be the key to structuring your class.

CREATE AN OUTLINE

What main points do you need to make to help them understand the topic you are teaching? Make a long list, then choose which points you feel are the most relevant to your audience.

For example: What things do you need to explain to help them recognize the importance of "cleaning with essential oils"?

Create a list of the points you feel will be most beneficial. For instance:

- What essential oils are
- How EOs naturally kills bacteria and germs
- Choosing suitable essential oils and where to buy them
- Using glass containers vs. plastic
- The importance of eliminating chemicals in the home

DEVELOP KEY OR MAIN POINTS

Find resources online and read books that can help build an outline and the key points of your main topic. For example:

What are Essential Oils?

- Essential oils are natural extracts that come from plants, which contain therapeutic and healing benefits. (name a few)
- Due to the distillation process, essential oils are potent. (make a comparison of how many pounds of rose petals to make oil)
- Essential oils contain chemical constituents from their specific plant. (name a few of the chemical names and their qualities)
- In a crude form, they were used by many ancient cultures for healing as opposed to today's over-the-counter medicine that comes with side effects. (offer a statistic of the number of deaths from prescribed drugs)

ASK QUESTIONS AND ENTERTAIN DISCUSSION

Include questions in your outline to build transition between main points or introduce or conclude the main point. This will bring the audience's attention back to the front. Plan for opportunities to let class members interact with you and others in the classroom. Never ask a question with an obvious answer (this can be insulting). Avoid questions with a "yes or no" answer that lead to no discussion. Instead, ask leading questions where they eagerly finish your sentence or an open-ended question. For example: "What products can you replace in your home right now with essential oils?"

REVIEW YOUR OUTLINE

Be sure to have a general timeline for how long each segment in your class will take. Make sure you have covered your main points. And don't forget to include facts and information to support your overall goal. For example: "Cleaning with essential oils can be just as effective compared to the chemicals found in most household cleaners without the harmful effects these products can do to our bodies, and our children. When used properly, essential oils will not cause any side effects like rashes, eye irritation, and respiratory damage." Some of the information you will want to include in every class is the therapeutic benefits of the oils, their safety information, the quality of the oils and GC/MS difference between perfume oils and a plant extracted essential oil, and dilution rates when blending (and discuss their concentration).

PREPARE FOR FAQS

Leave 10–15 minutes at the end of your class for questions from the audience. You will want to prepare for those "most frequently asked questions" in advance (have a cheat sheet ready just in case). Always keep eye contact with the person asking the question. Then, repeat the question for everyone else (every time). Why? You can use this to stall if you need to think about it. If you do not know the answer, ask the audience, "does anyone want to answer this?" Maybe say, "That is a good question. Let's get out the desk reference and look that up together."

CALL TO ACTION

When wrapping up your conclusion, tell them what you told them and what you want them to leave with. For example: "Today, we learned about the importance and benefits of cleaning with essential oils. I want to encourage you to start cleaning with essential oils. How many of you will make one new cleaning recipe this week and get rid of the cleaner that recipe replaces?"

PRACTICE, PRACTICE, PRACTICE

Go over the presentation at least three times before you teach your class. It is also helpful to make notecards or a PowerPoint presentation to help you stay on course. The more you can speak freely without struggling to look at notes, the better you connect with your audience.

FEEDBACK

Not only is the class a learning opportunity for your students, but each class also represents a learning opportunity for you. As you continue to gain experience in teaching, you will learn what works best for you and how to improve your classes moving forward. I highly suggest taking a little time after your class to reflect; the questions below are an excellent jumping-off point to get you started.

1. Did you accomplish the goal that you had for your class?
2. If not, how can you improve your class next time?
3. Did the people you wanted to attend the class come?

4. Did they take away from the class what you wanted them to?
5. Did you have enough time to prepare and set up for the class?
6. Were there any questions you were not prepared to answer from your knowledge or experiences?
7. Did you have all of the equipment you needed on hand for the class?
8. Was the classroom the right size for the class you hosted?
9. Did you create a way to contact those who attended to follow up on unanswered questions or let them know about future classes?
10. How can you improve your class in the future?

KEYS THAT UNLOCK YOUR CLASSROOM SUCCESS

Many people who have experience teaching classes or participating in an essential oil class agree on three primary keys for a successful course:

- Gain knowledge with experience on what you are teaching about.
- Keep your class focused on a specific, simple goal.
- Allow class members the opportunity to interact both with you and with the oils.

Other Things to Consider for Classroom Success

- Determine what you want to accomplish during the class.
- Make a plan for your class with that goal as the focus— and follow it.
- Keep it simple—don't try to teach everything at once.
- Have fun with what you are doing.
- Share your personal experiences.
- Interact with the people attending the class.
- Let your students interact with the essential oils as much as possible.

- Have books, handouts, and other information available for those who would like to learn more.
- Know (and be prepared to act on) all pertinent safety information for any essential oil you use during class.
- Don't try to fake what you don't know. It's okay to ask someone to look up something in a desk reference.

CHAPTER TWO SUMMARY

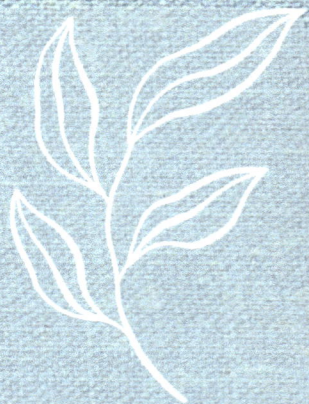

Brainstorming

- Who do you want to teach?
- How long of a class do you want to teach?
- Ideally, how many students would you like to have attend?
- What day of the week/time of the day do you want to hold your class?

Choosing Your Topic

- What topic in aromatherapy excites you?
- What do you know a lot about?
- What do your ideal students need to learn?

Choosing Your Essential Oils

- Essential oils used in your presentation should be easily accessible and affordable.
- What safety considerations might you have to take into account?
- What essential oils do you like? NEVER teach about an oil you don't have experience and a connection with.

Writing Your Lesson Plan

- Title / Description of your class
- Visual, auditory, and kinesthetic learning opportunities
- When / where are you holding your class?
- What essential oils are you teaching?
- What blending project are you teaching?
- What supplies do you need?
- What teaching tools do you plan to use?

Choosing a Blending Project

- What makes the most sense with the theme of your class?
- Will the venue you are using support the need for running a burner or any other equipment you might need?
- Is your project suitable for your ideal students?

Finding A Venue

- How big of a venue do you need?
- Public place or private home?
- Accessibility: wheelchair ramps, etc.?
- Are bathrooms easily accessible?
- Does the venue have the resources you need to teach your course effectively?

Teaching Tools

- Do you want to use PowerPoint?
- Do you need pictures you can share with students?
- Will you need a whiteboard to do any of your teaching with?
- Do you have videos or audio you want to share with your students?
- Are you going to use a course program?

Supplies

Think through every area of your class and determine what supplies you need to have on hand. Some examples:

- Scent Strips
- Essential Oils
- Carrier Oils
- Blending Containers
- Pens
- Extension Cords
- Computer, projector, etc.

Make a list of general supplies you will need for EVERY course, and then as you create classes, you can create add-on supply lists specific to what you are teaching.

Registering Students

- Do you want them to pre-register or just show up?
- What are you going to use to accept payment?
- Do you have a cancellation policy?
- Do you offer early-bird pricing?

Other Considerations

- Always take everything you need for a course with you—don't ever assume the venue will have what you need. If possible, set up a tote to be your mobile classroom and store all of your general supplies in it so you are ready to go whenever you need it.
- When creating a title for your course, inspire your pro-spective students to see it and think: "I HAVE to take that class."
- Remember to make your courses fluid—you can tweak and change things as you go and gain experi-ence teaching.

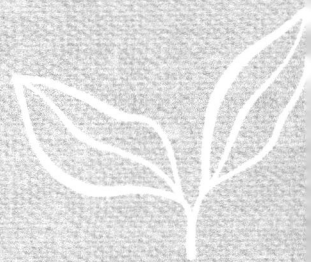

CHAPTER THREE

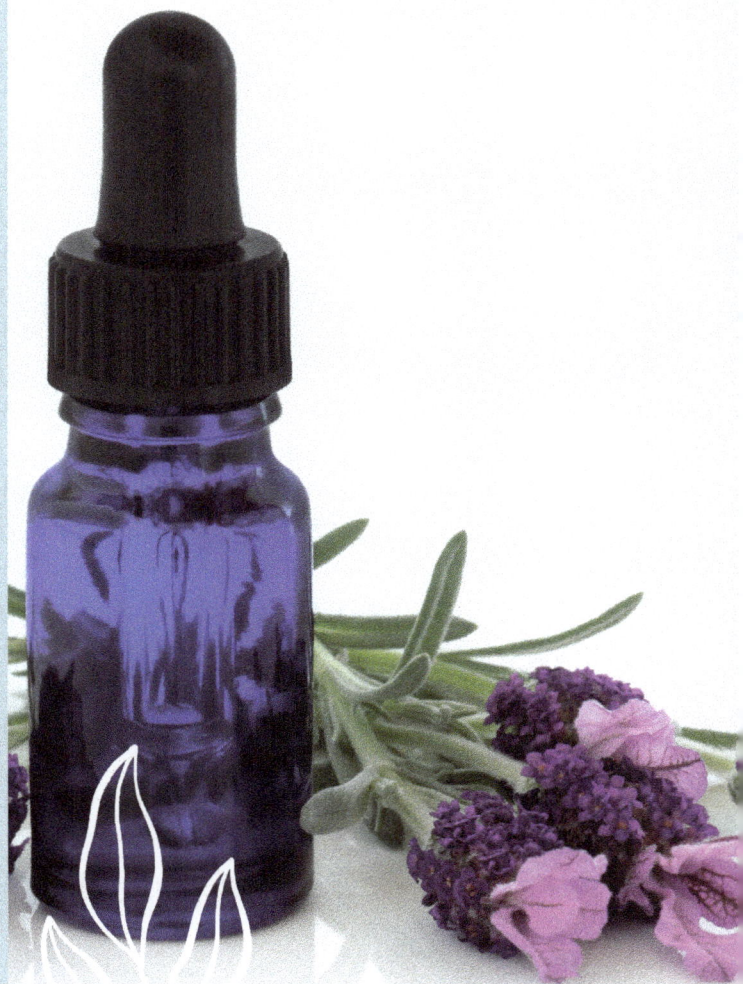

TEACHING AROMATHERAPY

This chapter will be talking about teaching topics specific to aromatherapy, including essential oils, blending, and dilution.

HOW TO TEACH ABOUT AN OIL

1. Announce the oil you are going to be talking about.
2. Place one drop of the essential oil on a perfume strip to pass around for students to inhale and experience. If you're conducting a small class, you may want to give each student their perfume strip to use. In larger classrooms, you can let people share. This will depend on the class and your objective.
3. As each oil is passed around, have each student open their manual to the datasheet for that oil and make notes of their thoughts on it.
4. Say both the common name and botanical name for the oil you are presenting. You may want to have it on a PowerPoint slide or even pre-record the name being spoken for people to hear if you are not confident saying it aloud.
5. Discuss the particulars about each oil: what part of the plant it came from, how it was distilled, the chemical family, etc.
6. When you share how the oil was distilled, tell why different methods are used to preserve the constituents of that oil.
7. Review the chart of the essential oil's therapeutic properties. Have students look up in the back of the manual terms they are unfamiliar with. Ask a student to read these aloud.
8. Discuss each oil's safety concerns and what they should be aware of when using it (i.e., phototoxicity).

9. Allow students to offer suggestions for how each oil could be used at home.

TEACHING A BLENDING PRODUCT

For some, this may come naturally; for others, it helps break down each step on making a product. When you begin teaching about your blending project, announce to the class what the project is and briefly go over the recipe you'll be using. With a class theme, you will remind students of the intention for the essential oil blend (i.e., this blend will help support the respiratory system). When choosing carrier oils, briefly explain why you chose the carriers you are using. This will help students understand the importance of carrier oils and how they have their beneficial properties as well. You will also want to explain why you chose the essential oils you're using.

In front of the room, demonstrate each step, walking students through step-by-step as you create the recipe together. At the same time, you will want to encourage good manufacturing practices such as wiping jars down with alcohol and so on. You will probably have stories to share as you explain why you're doing this (i.e., myrrh getting the top stuck).

Be sure to provide a copy of the essential oil recipe to each student. You will also want to provide blank labels and markers so each student can label their new product. Encourage each student to come up with a name for their product. After allowing ample time for each student to make their product, have a few people share what they named their product and how they plan on using it at home. This ensures they understand how to use it and why.

Steps to Teaching a Blend:

1. Announce to the class what the project is and briefly go over the recipe you'll be using.
2. Tell your students about the intention for the blend (i.e., this blend is helpful to support healthy respiratory function).
3. When it comes to carrier oils, explain why you chose the carriers you're using. This is an excellent way to introduce students to the idea that carrier oils have beneficial properties.
4. Explain why you chose the essential oils you're using.
5. Walk students step-by-step through creating the recipe you've chosen to make.
6. Teach good manufacturing practices—wiping jars down with alcohol, etc. Explain why you're doing this.
7. Provide a copy of the recipe to each student.
8. Provide each student with a label for their new product—allow them to name their product.
9. At the end of the blending session, have people share what they named their product and their intended use for the product.

SETTING UP A BLENDING STATION

Set up one set of blending materials for each student, along with a copy of the recipe. If you're making something such as a salve, you will oversee all of the hot plate work while explaining what you're doing.

TEACHING BLENDING

Explain to students what ingredients you're using and why. When it comes to essential oils, it's a good rule of thumb to allow the students only to use three different oils in their blend.

Explain the dilution for the product you're making.

Tell – Tell the students what their blend is to be used for (i.e., relaxation, pain, etc.).

Make – Make sure each student has a blank label to label their blend.

Let – Let students name their blends.

- Teach students good manufacturing practices for making products—keeping the space clean, sanitizing jars, etc. It's a good idea to lay a plastic or vinyl tablecloth on your workspace to make cleaning up easier—especially if you're in someone else's home or venue.
- Give students the number of drops of essential oil needed for the product, then let them decide how many drops of each oil they want to include.

AFTER BLENDING

Show – Show students how to clean up materials—if you can't show them, at least explain how to clean up.

Remind – Remind students to label their blends.

Talk – Talk a little more about the blend's benefits and give them ideas for using it.

COMMUNITY BUILDING AFTER BLENDING

To further build community after blending, go around the room and have students tell one another what they named their blend, what oils they used in their blend, and how they intend to use their blend. This will foster community building but also allows your students to learn from one another.

Make – Make sure your blending project is something students can easily repeat at home—the goal is to give them helpful information they can apply to their lives.

Keep – Keep blending projects safe—you don't want to use oils that have too many safety concerns.

Make at Home – Create blending kits that students can purchase and take home to use. This can be the same project you made in class or other similar projects.

FINDING RECIPES

While it's important that, as an aromatherapy teacher, you begin to create your own tried-and-true blends for projects, when you're starting or teaching something new, you may want to find recipes to use instead of making them.

Depending on the products you have selected to make during your class, you will want to find recipes to follow. In some cases, you will be making copies for each student to follow; in other cases, you may give the students guidelines with no limits to which oils to use and how many drops.

You may want to scan the internet, aromatherapy books, and magazines to find several product recipes to use for your class. Clip articles with recipes and save them in a pocket in the back of your notebook for future reference. Hint: In *Therapeutic Blending With Essential Oil by Rebecca Park Totilo,* you will find several "generic" recipes for numerous essential oil products. Use these as a guide. You will be able to choose which oils to use to make products.

BLENDING GUIDELINES

It's important to instruct your students in the proper way to handle essential oils. Here is a list of things to mention when teaching an essential oil class.

THE BIN (COFFEE BEANS, PERFUME STRIPS, LABELS, MARKERS, STIR RODS, OILS)

After you have introductions and have warmed up with an ice breaker, you will want to get everyone's attention again. Please go over the supplies in their bins, such as the coffee bean tin, perfume strips, labels, markers, essential oils, stir rods, etc. As you hold each item up, tell them how they will be using these in the class. During my live classes, I will have each student look at the supplies list form and essential oil list to check off all the items in their bin. You may want students to do another inventory at the end of class for longer classes to ensure essential oils or glass rods and bowls are all present and accounted for.

ORIFICE REDUCER

Most essential oils come with an orifice reducer eliminating the need for pipettes (but you might want to have a few glass droppers on hand, just in case). To ensure oils are not wasted, orifice reducers help prevent oil from coming out of the bottle too fast. Be sure to tell students not to touch these, if possible. You will need to demonstrate how to pour oil and show your students how to prevent touching the orifice with their hands.

WASHING HANDS

Be sure your classroom has access to a sink for washing hands and eyes if necessary. Remind students not to touch their eyes or other openings after handling essential oils. You will want to cover safety guidelines and safety tips during every class on properly handling essential oils and what to do if essential oils get into their eyes or on another sensitive area. Safety is important!

THE STRENGTH OF THE OILS

Many people are not aware of the potency of essential oils. If you can use a word picture (or PowerPoint slide) showing this, like stacking 80 teacups, one on top of another—so that they can see how many it would take to be equivalent to one drop of peppermint or lavender. That may not be realistic, but you could use the bottles example in another lesson shown or a PowerPoint slide demonstrating this as an example. Most people have the drugstore mentality that you need a spoonful to do the trick, but once they experience blending with essential oils, they will see just how powerful they are.

BLENDING DROP BY DROP

This is a SHOW DON'T TELL demonstration. Before students start their first blend, set up a small table in the front of the room and show students how to add one drop at a time to a blend (for example, in a bath salt). It's fairly simple to do: add one drop, stir, then smell it to see if it is something you like. As you already know, it's impossible to take a drop away, and when you add too much, you end up having to divide the blend up by making more product!

PERMISSION TO USE LESS

Even though you will be instructing your students in several blending techniques, including blending by notes, you will want them to know it's okay to use less! Certain essential oils should be used in lower doses, such as oregano, geranium, eucalyptus, etc.

HOW MANY OILS PER BLEND

Since most of your classes will be for beginners, you will want to encourage students to use only 3–5 oils per blend. Most blends tend to become "muddy" when too many fragrances are introduced.

DROP BY DROP METHOD

A popular method used in blending is called, Drop by Drop. With this technique, you will be taking time to become familiar with the oils and be learning as you go through all the steps. There is an old saying that says, follow the nose. In this case, you will be training your nose while creating your blend.

1. **Take out all of the essential oils you want to use in your blend and place them in front of you.** Be sure to have a container of coffee beans nearby to smell between oils to clear your palette (or nose). You will want to stop every few minutes to inhale the coffee beans or step outside to get fresh air.

2. **Take notes while creating your recipe blend.** Keep a notebook or use a form from your course to list all of the oils in your blend. As you add a drop of essential oil, place a tick mark next to that oil's name.

3. **Begin with one drop of oil (such as base note) that smells strongest to you.** After adding one drop of essential oil to your carrier oil, such as one ounce of jojoba, note what it smells like. This step is important in educating your nose as you learn to blend. All essential oils smell different once they are diluted.

4. **Next, add your middle note essential oil and pause to smell what these first two oils are like together.** You are training your nose in this teachable moment what these first two oils smell like when blended. If you want to adjust the aroma for future blends, knowing this can help you decide which oils to add to balance the scent perfectly.

5. **Continue adding a drop of the top note oil,** then pause to smell the new aroma.

6. **Once you have added one drop of each note, you can layer the blend** by adding different amounts of each oil.

7. **You will want to balance the oils' therapeutic properties (chemical constituents) with the blend's aroma.** When blending several oils, you will want to look for specific properties of different oils that you want to be strong in the blend, and in this case, you will add more of those oils.

8. **Once you reach your desired dilution or the blend smells perfect, you can stop.** Even if you intended on making a 2% dilution (12–18 drops) and you've added only nine drops and love the aroma, you can stop there. Or, if you want to add 14 drops in, that's okay too. The drop numbers are guidelines, not hard and fast rules.

9. **Stronger oils require fewer drops.** Use fewer drops of potent essential oils in your blend, such as floral oils (rose, jasmine, ylang ylang, and geranium). As you will soon discover, too many drops of certain oils may give you a headache. When using lighter oils, like the top notes citruses, you may want to add more, like 6 or 8 drops. This is because there are many more roses in one drop of rose oil than there are citrus peels in orange—so you will need to use less rose oil because of its concentration.

10. **Use fewer drops of oils high in ketones.** Essential oils such as peppermint and rosemary can be too stimulating for the nervous system and should be used in smaller quantities (approximately 3–5 drops).

HOW TO TEACH DILUTION

Essential oil dilution and safety are two concepts that are always associated with each other. You should never use an essential oil right from the bottle without prior dilution as this is very likely to cause irritated skin, among other side effects.

There are two main safety concerns associated with essential oils. The first one is avoiding skin reactions, while the other is avoiding systemic toxicity. Although skin reactions are immediately noticeable, systemic toxicities may go unnoticed for a long time, such as neurotoxicity, hepatoxicity, fetotoxicity, and carcinogenicity. You will want to advise your students of the importance of following safety guidelines to avoid such risks.

An essential oil should always be diluted with a carrier oil before applying it to the skin. The dilution ensures the essential oil will not evaporate right away, and as such, allow the oil's healing benefits enough time to soak into the skin. This also enables the essential oil to be applied over a larger surface area.

TYPES OF CARRIER OILS

Even though carrier oils are one of the main ways that you can use to dilute essential oils, there are many other options and alternatives. Other options include the use of butter, lotions, creams, conditioners, shampoos, aloe jellies, and castile soap as a means of diluting your essential oils. Additionally, most of the alternatives listed usually contain natural preservatives, making them ideal for your dilution and skincare needs.

DILUTION RATE FOR VARIOUS SCENARIOS

Accurate measurements are important as far as dilution is concerned. However, in a classroom setting, you may use drops which is not an exact measurement for demonstrating to your students. The dilution will also depend on the oil's viscosity and the size of the orifice reducer, and the rates presented here do not imply that each rate is safe for every situation or all essential oils.

1% DILUTION

This dilution is ideal for children who are aged two years and above. It is also suitable for long-term use, daily use, and facial applications. It also brings specific energetic effects of the oil to life, which is good for your skin health.

> 10 mL / 2 tsp = 3 drops
> 15 mL / 3 tsp / 1 tbsp = 4 drops
> 30 mL / 6 tsp / 2 tbsp / 1 oz = 9 drops

2% DILUTION

This rate is suitable for children, whole body products, and the regular use of oil daily. The rates are also acceptable and generally safe for children below ten years for treating spots. It is better to start on the low end and work your way up as you might require.

> 10 mL / 2 tsp = 6 drops
> 15 mL / 3 tsp / 1 tbsp = 9 drops
> 30 mL / 6 tsp / 2 tbsp / 1 oz = 18 drops

3% DILUTION

This rate is excellent for localized discomfort and application in a small area.

    10 mL / 2 tsp = 9 drops
    15 mL / 3 tsp / 1 tbsp = 13 drops
    30 mL / 6 tsp / 2 tbsp / 1 oz = 27 drops

5% DILUTION

This is a recommended rate for short-term use of essential oils for a period not exceeding two weeks.

    10 mL / 2 tsp = 15 drops
    15 mL / 3 tsp / 1 tbsp = 22 drops
    30 mL / 6 tsp / 2 tbsp / 1 oz = 45 drops

10% DILUTION

This rate is helpful for small areas of applications and in acute scenarios which require the essential oil.

    10 mL / 2 tsp = 30 drops
    15 mL / 3 tsp / 1 tbsp = 45 drops
    30 mL / 6 tsp / 2 tbsp / 1 oz = 90 drops

As a general rule, you should use a single drop of essential oil for every teaspoon of carrier oil to achieve a 1% dilution. For tricky scenarios, such as when you want to achieve a 0.50% dilution, you can increase the carrier oil you will be using since you cannot possibly measure half a drop. In cases where you cannot add carrier oil, you can round down your numbers to get how many drops of essential oil you will require. For instance, 2.5 drops would become 2 drops.

DILUTION FOR YOUNG CHILDREN

Children usually have thin and porous skin capable of absorbing anything that has been topically applied to it. On premature infants, essential oils are not recommended, but you can use the oil sparingly on full-term infants.

The dilution for these infants should be between 0.10% and 0.20%. This translates into 1-2 drops of essential oil for each ounce of carrier oil applied to the whole body.

You can also resort to 3-9 drops of the essential oil for each ounce of carrier oil when you need to apply the oil on specific spots. It is also vital to consult with a medical professional or a certified aromatherapist when using essential oils for children for a better decision.

Children between the age of 3 and 24 months should use a dilution of 0.25%-0.5%, while children between 2 and 6 years should use a general dilution rate of 1%-2%.

USING OILS NEAT

If a student insists on using an undiluted essential oil, encourage them first to seek advice from a certified aromatherapist. You can remind them that there are rare cases when applying the oils neat, such as to a bee sting or a sudden burn after touching a hot stovetop is appropriate. However, you will want to encourage them in safe usage for ongoing care to avoid developing skin sensitization or creating additional complications.

CONTRAINDICATIONS

Always ask students if anyone has epilepsy, asthma, or is taking prescribed medication; always seek advice from your physician before using essential oils. The same applies to people with a compromised immune system, pregnant and breastfeeding women, and anyone in doubt.

When applying essential oils, it always pays to play it safe to avoid adverse reactions. Ensure that your students use minimal dilution rates for effective results. You can always start with a patch test for safety and determine if the dilution rate you have chosen is safe for your skin.

DEMONSTRATING DILUTIONS

A way to show how strong essential oils is to show a 15ml bottle of essential oil next to a 750ml bottle of vegetable oil (same size as a bottle of wine). Then say to your class, "To properly dilute 300 drops (15ml bottle) essential oil at a 2% dilution rate would require an entire 750ml bottle of vegetable oil."

As we all know, dilution is an important part of using essential oils. Not only does diluting make the oil safe for application to the skin, but it also helps us to use less oil, making essential oils less costly.

There are several ways to demonstrate how to dilute a blend properly. Here is one example:

Use three bottles, one-ounce size. Use an essential oil bottle with an orifice reducer for this exercise, so you can show your students what it will look like when they're doing it themselves. If time allows during the blending portion of your class, allow your students to use your bottles of food coloring to count out drops as a practice run before making their products.

To demonstrate a 1% dilution with drops by counting out the drops using food coloring in a clear glass bottle that contains water. You will want to show the number of drops to add for top, middle, and base notes in different colors. For a 30-ml bottle, you will use nine drops total. For example, use two drops of red food coloring to represent the base note, three drops of blue food coloring to represent the middle note, and four drops of green food coloring to represent the top note.

You can adjust this exercise for any dilution rate. For a 2% dilution, you would use 18 drops of food coloring, and a 3% dilution would be 27 drops.

TOO MANY DROPS

When a student accidentally adds too many drops of oil, they will ask what to do. This will be a teachable moment for everyone in the class. Assist the student by showing how to divide the essential oil "juice" into another bowl or bottle (If possible, always add drops of essential oil to a clear glass bowl before adding to a carrier oil or final product bottle):

1. When too many drops come out, divide it up—split it up between two bowls and only use half of the essential oil blend for the final product.

2. If it is too strong, you can split the essential oil blend up with more lotion. Now, you will have two jars of lotion instead of one, for example.

You may want to give each student a copy of the following dilution chart to use for your class and at home when they're making their blends. This chart has been revised and may look different than most dilution rates in other courses and books. This update reflects the drop more accurately as 1.5 for a one-percent dilution instead of just one drop. However, it does pose a problem when trying to use 1.5 drops (since it is impossible to get a half drop from the bottle). Please remain flexible and let your students know that these are approximate measurements when using a dropper.

DILUTION RATE CHART

	5 ml	10 ml	15 ml	20 ml	25 ml	30 ml	50 ml	100 ml
.5%	.75	1.5	2.25	3	3.75	4.5	7.5	15
1%	1.5	3	4.5	6	7.5	9	15	30
2%	3	6	9	12	15	18	30	60
3%	4.5	9	13.5	18	22.5	27	45	90
4%	6	12	18	24	30	36	60	120
5%	7.5	15	22.5	30	37.5	45	75	150

You may also want to give examples of dilution rates and allow the students to use the chart to determine the correct number of drops for the blend.

Example 1: Say, "I want to make a 10 ml roller bottle with a 3% dilution; how many drops do I need?" (Answer: 9)

Example 2: Say, "I was making a blend and ended up using 150 drops—if I wanted to make it into a salve with a 5% dilution rate, how much salve would I need? (100 ml)

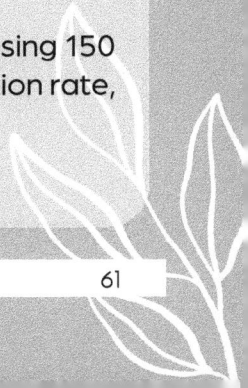

TEACHING ESSENTIAL OIL SAFETY

Safety is one of the most important topics to cover in your essential oil classes. You will want to cover both guidelines regarding essential oils in general and specific concerns for the oils you will be using in your class. You might consider going over each datasheet when you talk about each oil so that they can read along with you the therapeutic properties, safety concerns, etc. Of course, this will bring up several questions and concerns. Don't feel like you have to know all the answers. Bring a few good desk references with you and let students look through these for specific issues or concerns.

Note: You don't want to be overly cautious and cause new users to become scared to use oils. For the general population, essential oils are safe to use without any adverse side effects.

You will want to briefly cover each topic below and/or provide reading resources for students to look through regarding these subjects.

1. Essential oil dilution for topical use
2. Ingesting oils, "flavoring" their water
3. Oils that shouldn't be used around children
4. Oils that are unsafe for pets
5. Oils and potential interactions with medications
6. Phototoxicity
7. Sensitivity reactions

ESSENTIAL OIL SAFETY GUIDELINES

- Here are some guidelines you can go over with your students so they can achieve the maximum effectiveness and benefits.
- Avoid sunbathing, tanning booths, or using a sauna immediately after using essential oils.
- Be careful to avoid getting essential oils in the eyes. If you splash a drop or two of essential oil in the eyes, use a small amount of olive oil (or another carrier oil) to dilute the essential oil and absorb it with a washcloth. If serious, seek medical attention immediately.
- Take extra precautions when using oils with children. Never use undiluted essential oils on babies, and always store your essential oils out of reach from children.
- Never take essential oils internally unless advised by your medical practitioner or another qualified health professional.
- If a dangerous quantity of essential oil has been ingested, immediately drink olive oil and induce vomiting. The olive oil will help in slowing down its absorption and dilute the essential oil. Do not drink water—this will speed up the absorption of the essential oil.
- Most essential oils should be diluted before applying topically. Pay attention to safety guidelines—certain essential oils, such as cinnamon and clove bud, may cause skin irritation for those with sensitive skin. If you experience slight redness or itchiness, put olive oil (or any carrier oil) on the affected area and cover it with a soft cloth. Aloe vera gel also works well as an alternative to olive oil. Never use water to dilute essential oil—this will cause it to spread and enlarge the affected area. Redness or irritation may last 20 minutes to an hour.
- For sensitive skin or when using new oil, perform a "Skin

Patch Test." If irritation occurs, discontinue the use of such oil or blend. See the section on Skin Patch Test.

- If you are pregnant, lactating, suffer from epilepsy or high blood pressure, have cancer, liver damage, or another medical condition, use essential oils under the care and supervision of a qualified aromatherapist or medical practitioner.
- If taking prescription drugs, check for interaction between medicine and essential oils (if any) to avoid interference with certain prescription medications.
- To avoid contact sensitization (redness or irritation of the skin due to repeated use of same individual oil), rotate and use different oils.

WHAT CAN INFLUENCE THE SAFETY OF ESSENTIAL OILS?

QUALITY AND PURITY

It cannot be stressed enough that the purity of the essential oils to be used is paramount when it comes to safety considerations. Adulterated oils, in other words, essential oils blended with substances other than what they claim to be, can compound the potential risk of adverse reactions. Adulteration, a term frequently used in debates about one company's brand of oils being superior to another, is defined as "any practice that through intent or neglect, results in a variety of strength and/or purity."

NATURAL CHEMICAL COMPOSITION

Some oils contain naturally high levels of aldehydes and phenols, both compounds that can cause adverse reactions. Though all essential oils should be diluted to a safe concentration before being applied directly to the skin, products high in phenols or aldehydes should be used with even greater caution as they can be highly irritating. Products high in aldehydes include citronella and citral, sometimes in oils like melissa, lemongrass, mandarin, and lemon. Phenols are responsible for the scent of essential oils and can cause burning or corrosion of the skin when applied undiluted. Essential oils high in phenols include eucalyptus, rosemary, cinnamon, clove, thyme, oregano, and savory. Oils that contain either of these components should always be well diluted before topical application. Dilution rates vary and are usually between 3–5%, enough to eliminate any possibility of irritation.

METHOD OF DELIVERY SAFETY

There are three ways to use essential oils: diffused or inhaled directly, applied topically, and taken internally. Each method of delivery comes with its own set of caveats and safety considerations.

Inhalation, whether directly, vaporized, or by diffusion, represents a very low-risk factor for most individuals. Even in close quarters, the concentration levels will rarely reach a point where they pose a serious threat. A case could be made to avoid prolonged exposure to highly concentrated levels of any essential oil vaporized continuously into a closed space for an hour or more. The individual may experience nausea, headaches, and other adverse effects.

If **ingested internally**, consider that essential oils are concentrated thousands of times over from the raw material. For instance, it may take more than a ton of oregano to make one pound of essential oil, so consuming unnaturally large amounts of it would probably not be a good idea. While several essential oils may be listed as GRAS (generally regarded as safe), most essential oils are not safe for internal use, and those that are should be used only with extreme caution. Ingestion should be restricted to acute cases only, much like pharmaceutical preparations, and only ingested under the supervised guidance of a qualified practitioner. There isn't a one-size-fits-all for a maximum dosage of a particular oil with so many other considerations that must be factored in, such as a person's general health, age, possible drug interaction with prescribed medication, and duration of use.

Many essential oils that boast antibacterial, antifungal, and antioxidant properties could cause an imbalance in someone's gut bacteria and could potentially cause great harm if misused or overused in this way. Several organizations, including the Alliance of International Aromatherapists (AIA) and the National Association for Holistic Aromatherapy (NAHA), have clear guidelines regarding the internal use of essential oils and believe that the use of undiluted or internal use of essential oils should only be advised by a trained aromatherapist with an appropriate level of education including chemistry, basic physiology, and anatomy, consultation practices including diagnostics, and formulation techniques and safety practices regarding each specific internal route (oral, vaginal, or rectal). Please visit AIA's website http://www.alliance-aromatherapists.org/aromatherapy/aromatherapy-safety/ for more information.

If used **topically**, either in a skin preparation, massage oil, or for any other reason, the essential oil should be diluted sufficiently to reduce the risk of irritation. A 3–5% solution translates roughly to 3–5 drops per teaspoon (5 ml) of carrier oil. Different guidelines apply when using on children, babies, or pregnant women. Never use an essential oil full strength on the skin, and test dilutions on a small area, if possible, to ensure safety. Some oils are phototoxic, making the skin more sensitive to UV light and potentially leading to blisters, burns, and discoloration with even moderate exposure to the sun. Phototoxic oils include all citrus oils: grapefruit, lemon, orange, bergamot, and lime. Some distillation methods can reduce the phototoxic nature of these oils, but the user should always err on the side of caution, no matter what the claim.

STRENGTH AND CONCENTRATION

Dilution factors for most essential oils are between 1% and 5%. At this strength, there are relatively few safety concerns. The more concentrated the blend becomes, the greater the potential for an adverse reaction. Essential oils are lipophilic in nature, meaning that they are fat-soluble and stored in the body for a period of time, presenting a greater potential for irritation. Other factors that should be considered include the area of the skin to be treated as well as the client's sensitivities or intolerances.

SKIN QUALITY

If the skin is damaged in any way, infected, or inflamed, it may be more susceptible to irritation. It is not recommended to use essential oils on damaged or broken skin, as the skin may absorb far more than would be safe even under normal circumstances. Adverse reactions are more likely to occur, and the skin condition may become worse. Use extreme caution with clients who are observed to have damaged skin.

AGE OF THE INDIVIDUAL

For use on children and babies, the concentrations should be reduced accordingly. Children have a heightened sensitivity to essential oils, and some should be avoided entirely. These include wintergreen, peppermint, rosemary, eucalyptus, and birch. The aging skin may also be more sensitive to essential oils, so greater dilution factors should be considered in their case as well.

AROMATHERAPY BLENDS FOR CHILDREN

When we think of creating therapeutic blends with essential oils for kids, there are several potential uses and benefits for children. Although aromatherapy is beneficial for people of all age groups, it is ideal for treating common ailments children may experience. In addition, children will enjoy the aromas of essential oils and connect them to positive feelings. Moreover, the therapeutic blend of oils used in aromatherapy is natural and does not have any adverse effects compared to the medicines used to treat diseases in conventional medicine.

Other ways in which essential oils are beneficial for your children include helping them relax, improve their digestion, strengthen their immune health, and create a general balance and harmony in their bodies. Of course, essential oils are not medicines, nor are they meant to replace medication. As an aromatherapist, our objective with recommending essential oils for children and adults alike is to help the body and mind attain a state of homeostasis, thereby decreasing sickness.

Precautions When Using Essential Oils With Children

- Be aware of the chemical components within the essential oils you use in your therapeutic blend for kids. Some oils may contain large amounts of a citrus component or a potent herbal extract that may cause an allergic reaction in children.
- It is best to test for allergic reactions in your kids before using any particular oil or therapeutic blend on them. Be sure to do a skin patch test to check for any allergic reaction.
- According to Medline Plus, applying lavender oil to the skin of young boys who have still not reached the stage of puberty is unsafe. This is due to the hormone-like effects of lavender essential oil that could cause an adverse effect on the normal hormonal balance. Using lavender has resulted in developing a condition called gynecomastia, which is characterized by abnormal breast growth in boys.
- Aromatherapy use is not recommended for children less than six months of age.
- Aromatherapy is not meant to substitute professional medical attention when needed.
- Use the best quality oils available for making your therapeutic blends so you will get the best results.
- Never allow a child to use an essential oil without supervision.

In addition to the considerations mentioned above concerning the safe use of essential oils, the following general guidelines should be followed:

- Avoid the application of essential oils on allergic or inflamed skin
- Avoid undiluted application
- Avoid application to open wounds or otherwise damaged skin
- Dilute appropriately with a carrier oil before applying
- Perform skin patch tests, especially if sensitivity is already known

SKIN PATCH TEST

Certain essential oils can cause sensitization or an allergic reaction in some individuals. When using a new oil for the first time, you may want to perform a simple skin patch test on the inside of your arm or your chest. Place one drop of the essential oil into a carrier oil. Apply one drop on the skin and cover with a bandage.

If skin becomes irritated and red, remove the bandage and immediately wash the area with soap and water. If, after 12 hours, no irritation has occurred, it is safe to use on the skin.

SENSITIZATION AND ALLERGIC REACTIONS

Many may wonder if it is possible to be allergic to pure essential oils. And, the answer is yes.

Sensitization is defined as the exposure to an allergen that results in the development of hypersensitivity according to the Miller-Keane, Encyclopedia, and Dictionary of Medicine, Nursing, and Allied Health. Hypersensitivity is, in a sense, an allergic reaction, which Farley Medical Dictionary (2012) defines "as a local or general reaction of an organism following contact with a specific allergen to which it has been previously exposed and sensitized; immunologic mechanisms gives rise to inflammation or tissue damage."

Any essential oil can become an allergen by using undiluted on the skin, including popular oils such as lavender or tea tree. So, while some essential oils carry precautions and have a reputation for being a potential allergen or possibly cause sensitization, any essential oil used neat (undiluted) can set the individual up for a possible reaction, which causes them to become allergic to that essential oil forever.

There are four types of allergic reactions, but only two are relevant to aromatherapy or essential oil usage. According to Robert Tisserand, author of Essential Oil Safety, delayed hypersensitivity accounts for 90% of allergic reactions. The other type of allergic reaction is immediate hypersensitivity (generally not anaphylactic) which accounts for the other 10%. Of course, not all oils do cause such reactions, but certainly, the risk is still there. The less you dilute your blend, the more likely you are at risk for developing sensitization. As you begin to work with the oils, you will quickly learn those more likely to cause reactions (such as cinnamon or cassia).

DETERMINING AN ADVERSE EFFECT

Is breaking out with a rash or noticing redness after applying essential oils an adverse effect, or is the body just detoxing? You will hear this frequent question as more people experiment with essential oils but are unaware of their potency and safe usage.

First, define "adverse effect" when using an essential oil or essential oil blend. Any unpleasant effect that you were not expecting could be considered an adverse effect. The Aromatherapy United website (http://aromatherapyunited. org) describes it as any reaction to an essential oil that was not intended could be viewed as an adverse effect. These effects can range from minor and discomforting to much more severe and permanent.

Some examples of adverse effects are (dependent on the type of oil applications: topical, oral, inhalation):

- Redness
- Rashes
- Blistering
- Itching
- General Irritation
- Chemical Burning
- Pigmentation Changes
- Headache

- Nausea
- Interferes with medication
- Alters blood pressure
- Bleeding
- Sores
- Numbness
- Tingling
- Nerve deadening

If you have experienced any kind of adverse reaction from essential oil use or someone you know has, the Atlantic Institute of Aromatherapy is collecting data to help ensure safe practices. Please take a moment and fill out an Injury Report Form at: http://atlanticinstitute.com/injury-reporting/.

TEACHING HOW TO MAKE BODY LOTION

You will want to instruct your students in the proper way to make a cream or body lotion and share some of the information below so they know the difference. Use these questions as prompts of what to mention in class.

- What are the things you need to tell your students about lotions and creams? Is there a difference between a cream or body lotion?
- Are the blending dilutions the same as for other products? (lotions have higher water content and are non-greasy and lighter than cream).
- What happens if you use dark oils? Will it change the color of your lotion?
- What is the dilution rate for a cream? (Hint: 2% dilution)
- Any concerns? Phototoxicity, skin irritation?
- What about different amounts of drops based on the oil itself (such as intense, concentrated florals like jasmine, geranium, ylang ylang)?

When it comes to understanding the distinction between body lotion and body cream, the combination of oil and water is very important. Any type of moisturizer has its own particular composition and its own unique set of benefits. Body lotion and cream are used to avoid dryness and cracked skin; both will comfort and moisturize. Perhaps the most significant difference between lotion and cream is that lotion has higher water content. Lotion is typically is lighter weight than cream and is non-greasy. Creams are thicker in consistency than lotions and provide a barrier that keeps skin ultra-hydrated. Lotions and creams contain both an oily agent with a watery agent. Both assist in replenishing the oil in the skin and also protect against loss of moisture.

BODY CREAM

Body cream is more substantial and contains a higher viscosity or pasty mixture of water and oil. Creams penetrate the skin and give a barrier that stops more moisture loss than lotion. Creams, though, often feel greasier. The amount of water and oil in cosmetic cream and lotion differs, which is also affected by other ingredients, such as paraffin oil. Considering body cream is heavier, it is usually available in a tub or jar container.

BODY LOTION

Body lotions usually are not as sticky, and the skin more easily absorbs them. This kind of moisturizer usually has greater water content, can be found in a bottle, and may also be poured out in a liquid form. A lotion is best for skin that is not extremely dried out or when it's preferable not to have a wet, oily feeling on the skin.

TEACHING HOW TO USE CARRIER OILS

Using a carrier oil is a big part of blending. Your students will probably ask you what a carrier oil is. In the simplest terms, they are fatty vegetable oils composed of bigger molecules that offer the necessary lubrication and moisture to the skin. While most consider carrier oils as just a vehicle for applying essential oils to the skin, they offer their own healing properties that essential oils do not possess. Your students will discover how much more their aromatherapy experience is enhanced by choosing the best carrier to use with their essential oils. You will want to instruct your aromatherapy students in the proper way to use carriers and share with them the differences in each. Be sure to bring several choices so students can experiment with each carrier oil and learn about their benefits.

- What things do you need to tell your students about a carrier oil? Does it have a shelf life?

  A carrier oil's shelf life, which is the length of time before a particular oil begins to turn rancid, can be significantly influenced by heat and light. You will want to tell your students to store their oils in a cool, dark place to preserve their freshness and, in some cases, refrigerate as heat and sunlight can shorten their shelf life. When refrigerating, oils may appear cloudy but will regain their clear state upon returning to room temperature. If you have a large amount of carrier oil on hand, you can freeze the unused portion until ready for use.

- Does the number of drops of essential oil used in a blend change when using a carrier oil?

  When you use essential oils for a massage, you will need to dilute with a carrier oil. Generally, two drops of therapeutic grade essential oil should be used per teaspoon of carrier oil (follow individual recipes when available). A full body massage takes about one to two ounces of carrier oil. Any natural carrier oil (except mineral oil) is acceptable to use when preparing a massage blend. Add 12–18 drops of essential oil to 30 ml of carrier oil as a general rule. For children and the elderly, use only 6–9 drops of essential oil to 30 ml of carrier oil.

TEACHING HOW TO MAKE INHALERS

These portable inhalers let you breathe in essential oils. They are great for treating sudden symptoms of anxiety and stress. They are also beneficial for respiratory issues and can unblock your airways so you can breathe freely. These are great for carrying on you when you need a mood lift, clear sinus congestion, or if a wave of nausea hits. Because they are compact, you can use these anywhere. Making an essential oil inhaler or aromatherapy inhaler stick is quite simple and can be used for multiple issues such as anxiety, colds, and flu remedies for children to take to school or on trips in a car or airplane.

Inhalers are super easy to make! Blank inhalers come in four pieces for making aromatherapy inhalers: the cap (bottom), the inner tube with the hole on top, the cover, and the cotton wick. Essential oil inhalers do not need a carrier such as vegetable oil for dilution. The cotton wick holds the essential oil in place. You only need to add about 15 drops of your essential oil blend.

Essential oil inhalers are safe for kids to take to school (especially when they have the sniffles). They are also great for travel to help with jet lag, motion sickness, or sleep aid after a long flight.

You will want to demonstrate how to use the inhaler correctly.

The best way to use it is to place the inner tube (cap removed) next to your nostril while pinching your other side closed and breathing deeply. You can also use the inhaler by placing it in your mouth while closing your lips around it and breathing deeply to get the essential oil vapors into your lungs.

These inhalers last for months and can prevent symptoms from getting worse. They are called personal inhalers because they are used with essential oils safe for inhalation to meet their individual needs. Please be sure to check essential oil safety guidelines for more usage information. You can advise your students to use as needed, which is usually once or twice a day.

This is an easy and fun activity for students of all ages to make. Use these questions to help you prepare for this activity before class.

- Are there any blending dilutions necessary with this product? (Hint: use only 15–18 drops of essential oils, undiluted or neat)
- Important: Use different amounts of drops based on the essential oil you are using (such as intense, concentrated florals like jasmine, geranium, ylang ylang, etc.)
- Which essential oils should not be used in an inhaler?
- Are there any concerns?
- Please talk about the convenience of carrying them in their purse or pocket. Storage? Keeps up to a year (maybe longer).

TEACHING HOW TO BLEND WITH BATHS SALTS

Aromatic baths are a fantastic natural alternative to modern medicine when treating common ailments and mood swings. Salts for the bath alone have many therapeutic properties. The most popular salts come from the Himalayas, the Dead Sea, the Pacific Ocean, the Mediterranean Sea, and the Great Salt Lake in Utah, USA. Each kind plays a particular role in the health of our body and skin.

Epsom salt is commonly used as a bath salt and has many benefits, such as reducing the prune look of skin. Because the salt changes the osmotic balance of the bathwater, it allows your skin to absorb more water. Magnesium sulfate, one of the main components in bath salts, has anti-inflammatory properties that help the body stay healthy by avoiding a cellular breakdown. Phosphates, which are also found in bath salts, soften the skin and calluses, helping to exfoliate the skin and keep it smooth.

Diseases such as psoriasis and atopic dermatitis are treated with high sea salt concentrations in water; this is why many people with these and other skin ailments go to the Dead Sea for therapy. Other physical benefits from sea salts include stimulating natural circulation, relief from athlete's foot, removing corns and calluses, and relaxation of tense and aching muscles. Rheumatism, arthritis, and chronic lower back pain can be cured with high sea salt concentrations in water.

You will want to instruct your aromatherapy students in the proper way to use bath salts as a carrier for the bath and know about their differences. It's always fun to bring several varieties of salts such as Dead Sea, Himalayan, Hawaiian Salt, Epsom, etc., so students can experiment with each one and learn about their benefits. Answer these questions below as prompts to consider when teaching your aromatherapy students about using bath salts.

- What are the blending dilutions when using essential oils in the bath or as a scrub? (Hint: blend salts at 1% dilution)
- Are there any essential oils you should not use in the bath? What about the number of drops based on the oil itself, like intense oils?
- How much should you use in one bath? (Hint: About an ounce)
- Are there any concerns when using oils in the bath? Phototoxicity, skin irritation?

TEACHING HOW TO MAKE SPRAYS

You will want to instruct your students in the proper way to make a linen, room, or body spray. Use these questions as prompts to determine what things you need to tell your students about sprays.

- Are the blending dilutions the same for the linen spray, room, and body or facial spray?
- What do we do differently for a room spray versus a body spray? What about specific oils?
- Any concerns? Phototoxicity, skin irritation?
- What about thick oils in a spray bottle?
- How do you get the water and oil to mix?

LINEN SPRAYS

Linen spray in a spray bottle provides a fine mist of the essential oil product to be sprayed over linens, towels, sofa cushions, clothes, and carpets. It's used to refresh linens and soft furniture between washes, or it's sprayed onto a cloth to use when ironing to provide a pleasing and good scent to clothing. Linen spray could be used on apparel when ironing to give your clothes a gentle and permanent perfume. Your clothes that are not dirty but have been worn in a smoky atmosphere could be refreshed by spraying them with linen spray and hanging them outside. And it also works to refresh clothes that have been dry-cleaned or even hand-washed, allowing more time between washes.

Linen spray can be used on sheets and pillows to pass on a fresh, fragrant scent between washes. Linen sprays have essential oils that could be used in the bedroom in this manner before resting, with a variety of aromatherapy benefits. The fragrances of different kinds of essential oils can have a soothing, calming, or bodily effect, such as how the scent of lavender is known to help sleepiness.

Fabric cushions and carpets could be spritzed with linen spray to refresh them and to make them have a pleasing fragrance in the room. Linen spray is mainly helpful for furniture and cushions that can't be removed for cleaning or aren't always clean. This could be especially helpful if you are trying to sell your home, as prospective buyers will be pleased with the smell of your home.

Linen spray could be used similarly as an air freshener by spraying into the air to give a pleasing fragrance to the entire room. This is helpful when guests visit at short notice and do not have time to carefully clean and air out your rooms.

When traveling, you can spray on linen and use it on hotel beds to give a pleasant scent. This could also be useful for those who have a problem sleeping in a strange bed as it provides a bodily reminder of home. If you're given a smoking room, spray can also help mask the horrible smell when sprayed on the curtains and carpets as well as into the air.

ROOM SPRAYS

A room spray is a type of diffusion that quickly releases a more concentrated amount of oil into the air. You will use approximately 30–40 drops of essential oil with hydrosol or mineral water and vodka if hydrosol is unavailable. Use as needed to deodorize or fumigate a room or create a special atmosphere. Room sprays are incredibly convenient for disinfecting an area, such as a sickroom, or repelling insects.

If creating a room spray, you may want to use a hydrosol (floral water), to which you can add the essential oils for designing a room spray. To ensure the essential oils disperse throughout the hydrosol or another water–based carrier (and stay mixed), you will need to add an additional product called "solubol," an all–natural dispersant. If this is not available, you may substitute aloe vera or glycerin in its place.

Room sprays are great for changing the mood of a room. You may choose any fragrant hydrosol or floral water to use as your base. Typically a 2–ounce room spray calls for 40–50 drops of essential oil, depending on the aromatic strength of your oils. When using a hydrosol as the carrier, you can use fewer drops of essential oil.

TEACH HOW TO PRONOUNCE LATIN NAMES

On most essential oil bottles, the Latin name is listed below the common name. You will want to make sure you know how to pronounce the Latin botanical names correctly, so you are confident in teaching your students how to say them. If you only have a few oils, you can slowly say each name with them.

Be sure to write out the phonetic spelling of each word in your notes (spell it as it sounds), so you won't stumble over the name when reading through your notes. To become familiar with the Latin names, practice each one ahead of the class.

DEMONSTRATING HOW TO MAKE A PRODUCT

In your class, you will want to show your students how to make a product. Use these steps as a guideline.

1   Tell them the intention of your product. For example, "Today, we are going to make a skin lotion."

2   Do a demonstration of getting the lotion from the container (hopefully, it has a pump). This may mean each student will need to go up to the front and use the dispenser to get the lotion out (if in a large container) or a small bottle of lotion that can be passed around.

3   Remind them of the dilution rate. Ask them how many drops you'll need (let them do the math). State that this is a 2-ounce bottle or tub, so how many drops would you use in that? (Answer: 10–12 drops)

4   Write on a whiteboard or prepare a PowerPoint slide showing dilution rate, then ask how many drops again.

5   Choose three oils using the perfume strips they made. Then decide how much of each oil to use. Ask the class how much of each oil to use.

6   Demonstrate the Drop-by-Drop Method.

7   When using thick oils, you will want to talk about the viscosity of those oils. Show how some don't want to come out of the bottle. Offer recommendations for what to do when the oil is stuck, such as running under hot water or rolling between your hands.

8   Show students how to make a label for their product. The bin you provide should have pens, labels, and containers for each student.

9   Depending on the label you provide, you might want to have a clear piece of tape to protect the writing of the product.

10   Ask for questions and check to make sure everyone understands how to make the product.

CHAPTER THREE SUMMARY

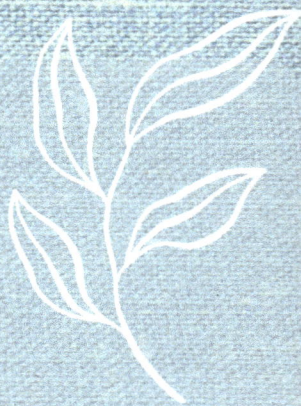

A short class is a great way to introduce new people to the wonderful world of essential oils. During this workshop, you'll have enough time to teach a few oils and create an essential oil blend or product—allowing students to apply what they've learned.

Be organized and stay on track with your class schedule. One hour isn't a lot of time to do a class, so you'll want to make sure you're maximizing every minute.

You will want to use 3-6 oils for a one or two-hour class. For a one-hour class, you might only have time for a lecture and pass around a few oils for the attendees to smell. For a two-hour class, you can bring about six oils to have people smell and talk about. Depending on the length of your lecture, you may have time for one blending product. For a three-hour class, you can make two blends. Here are some tips to consider and information to have on hand:

TEACHING TIPS TO REMEMBER

- Talk for 10-15 minutes to get across the general information before you start to pass around the oils (at this point, they will be half-listening and miss important information).

- Have people smell a few of the oils in the whole group, then, if appropriate, have them break into small groups smell the oils. Ask the attendees what body system each oil would be good for based on its smell.
- Pose a few questions to the group, such as if they have ever used oils before, share any good stories about them, what the smells remind them of, and so on.
- When talking about the oils, pass them around for each person to smell (use labeled perfume strips instead of smelling out of a bottle).
- Whenever possible, demonstrate how to make an essential oil blend.
- Be sure to balance lecture and student participation, question and answer time, smelling oils, and making blends.
- Always include visual tools (books, magazines, pictures, and websites).

INFORMATION TO INCLUDE IN EVERY CLASS

- Safety information
- Therapeutic benefits of the oils covered in class
- Purity of essential oils and the GC/MS (how to know the difference between perfume oils and a plant-extracted essential oil—ALWAYS DO THIS!)
- Dilution rates for blending
- Information on other classes you will be teaching

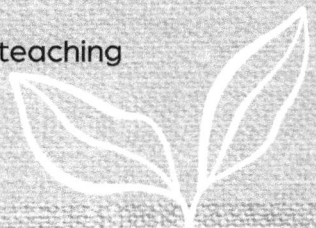

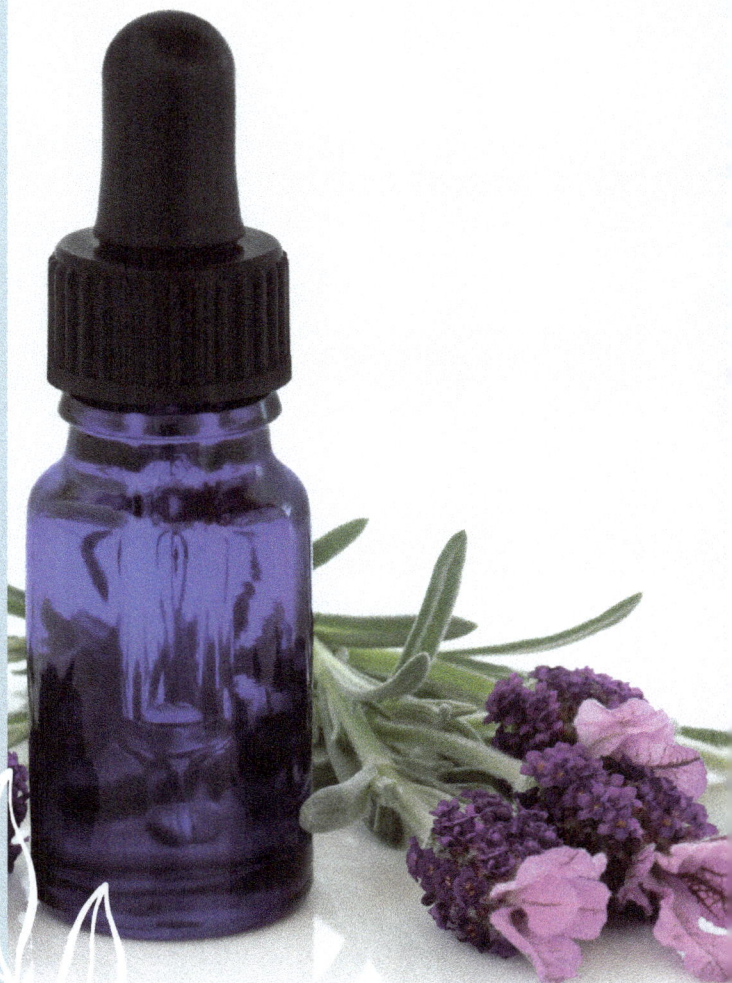

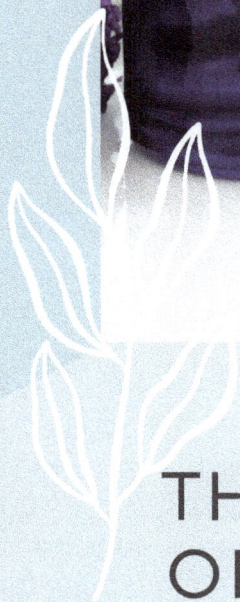

THE BUSINESS OF TEACHING AROMATHERAPY

Teaching can be a lucrative part of your existing aroma-therapy practice, or it can be a stand-alone business for you. Like any other business, a lot goes into running a teaching business, including pricing your classes and marketing.

General Teaching Business Tips:

1. Treat your teaching business like a business
2. Create a business entity for yourself—this can be as simple as a "doing business as" designation.
3. PayPal is a great, low-cost way of collecting tuition from students. Other options include Stripe or Square.
4. Look into getting liability insurance—some venues may require you to have this, plus it covers you if someone gets injured during one of your classes.

HOW MUCH TO CHARGE

Determining what you want to be paid is one of the most important things to consider. It is not simply how much you have invested in supplies, but also your TIME is of value. Everyone has a different idea of what is a fair price for an event. One rule of thumb could be to charge approximately $20 per hour per student.

So, let us say you are teaching a two-hour First-Aid with Essential Oil class; you can charge between $40-50 for the entire event. Of course, other costs such as location/rent and added expenses for oils and handouts must be factored in. You will want to check around to see what competitive businesses charge for similar classes. Your time and expertise is something that should not be devalued or given away. You are offering a very specialized class, and most people understand this.

You're going to want to consider all of the costs of holding your course—both indirect and direct costs. The first, most important question you need to ask is what you want or need to make at the end of the class. Teaching a class takes work, and you deserve to be paid for that work.

Next, you're going to want to look at what the community you're planning to teach in will pay for a class. A way to figure this out is to look at courses that others hold in your area (fitness classes, wellness classes, etc.) and see what they're charging. If you see them only holding one class and then never having another, it's a good indication that they didn't get much interest in the course; the price could be a factor in that interest level.

You're looking for a sweet spot when it comes to pricing your class. You want to make enough that you're happy with what you're making, where people will see the value in attending, and where the price won't turn people off. It's a good idea to know what you will want to charge for classes down the road for future events. This way, when you host your first event, you can offer an "introductory price" and leave some wiggle room to slowly increase your price as your skills get better and your audience grows.

In determining what to charge for a class, you will need to figure out your expenses, including the costs involved in making each product. The first thing you will want to do is calculate the price of a product.

COSTS TO CONSIDER

- Your time and travel expenses
- Essential oils
- Bottles and containers
- Labels
- Rent
- Bins to hold the oils and supplies
- Markers for the student blends
- Glass stir rods
- Whiteboard or chalkboard
- Paper towels
- Advertising
- Snacks

ADVERTISING AND MARKETING

These days, there are a lot of ways to advertise your class. You can follow the traditional methods of a standard local newspaper, radio, and press releases to television stations. You will also want to include social media and Google Adwords.

Some important thoughts as you're thinking about your marketing plan:

1. Create a brand for your classes—make people remember you.
2. Make sure when advertising the classes that you make it known that the tuition price includes a product.
3. Give the product they'll be making a value, "You're going to leave with a customized (type of product)—a value of $___."
4. Create excitement around your course.
5. Create a sense of scarcity— "Only four seats available!"

Reaching Your Audience

- Email Mailing List
- Letter to Students (manual letter)
- Professional Organizations
- Fiverr.com (for getting a press release out)
- Elance (hire a marketing manager)
- Blogs
- Google advertising
- Website

PLACES TO ADVERTISE

- Facebook
- Google Adwords
- NAHA Listing (members only)
- DoTerra Wellness Advocates
- Young Living Distributors
- Recreational Centers
- Health Food Stores
- Libraries
- Chamber of Commerce
- Local Fresh Markets
- Network Marketing
- Referral Program
- Joint Venturing
- Local Spas

It is important to get the word out. Even though this is one of the areas most people ignore, it is one of the most important ways to spend your time, energy, and money!

- Start a Google Paid Ad about one or two months before the event
- Start a Facebook Paid Ad about a month before the event
- Use and follow Hyperalerts.com
- Spend 15 minutes every morning with Facebook adding posts (space them out in time)
- Blog once a week (more often if you are just getting started)
- Use an email service such as Mailchimp.com to build a free mailing list and send out a notice about your upcoming class
- Use Constant Contact or another service if you want to

set up an autoresponder program where emails are sent out automatically when a person signs up for your email list and gets an email according to your specifications

- Hire a marketing manager on Fiverr.com to help you get the word out (post a press release in the news feed of major newspapers and websites)
- Try Canva.com or PicMonkey.com (pictures with words)
- Connect with your local Holistic Chamber of Commerce
- Join Professional Organizations: NAHA, AIA
- Use Twitter (add a couple of tweets a day)
- Post on Pinterest
- Post YouTube Videos
- Hang flyers at your local library
- Hang flyers at your local health food store, whole foods market, etc.
- Create a Facebook event page
- Create an Eventbrite event
- Have postcards created with the course information on it to leave on local bulletin boards

DEVELOPING YOUR ELEVATOR PITCH

Your elevator pitch is a short blurb that you can use when someone asks what you do or asks more about your class or aromatherapy. Take your time to get elevator pitches down for the following topics—practice them on a friend or family member and have them ready the next time you're asked. Keep your elevator pitches to no more than 30 seconds—you're not looking to teach them everything you know, just enough to pique their interest and want more information.

1. What is aromatherapy?
2. What is an essential oil?
3. What do you do?

HOLDING FREE CLASSES AS MARKETING

Hosting a short, free event can go a long way to getting your name out there and helping your audience grow.

What you will need for a free event:

1. Three inexpensive oils
2. Perfume strips
3. Email list sign-up
4. Short blurbs about aromatherapy

When you're talking with people at the event, give them a scent strip with a drop of essential oil on it to smell, chat with them a little about aromatherapy, and have them sign up for your email list. When you send out emails about upcoming classes, you can send these people an invitation also. Free events are a great way to grow your email list audience for very little expense.

Once a student signs up for your class, you will want to send a follow-up letter containing all the pertinent information about the class. Be sure to include a map and/or directions to the class location.

CHAPTER FOUR SUMMARY

Business Basics

Create – Create a business entity—this can be as simple as a DBA "doing business as" name.

Check – Check into liability insurance—you want to be covered if someone gets injured during one of your classes; some venues may require proof of insurance for rentals.

Treat – Treat your business like a business.

Pricing Your Class

- How much do you want to make for each course?
- Keep track of supply costs—use this to determine your cost of holding the class
- Don't forget to include rental fees into your costs
- What's the sweet spot? That spot where you're making money and students aren't shying away from signing up due to the price.

Marketing

Spread the word about your class locally and online:

- Social Media
- Community bulletin board
- Local publications
- Flyers
- An incentive for student referrals
- Joint ventures

The Elevator Pitch

Develop these mini speeches; memorize them, practice them, and have them ready at all times. Prepare 15-30 second explanations for the following:

- What you do
- What you teach
- What aromatherapy is
- What essential oils are

Additional Ways to Make Money by Teaching

- Offer one-on-one consultation for students
- Purchase extra supplies and create blending kits for students to purchase and take home
- Sell oils by the drop during your class
- If you make products, include information on your products in your course materials
- Create a short ebook that you can market during your class

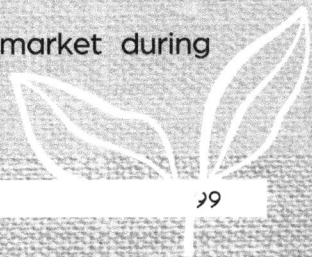

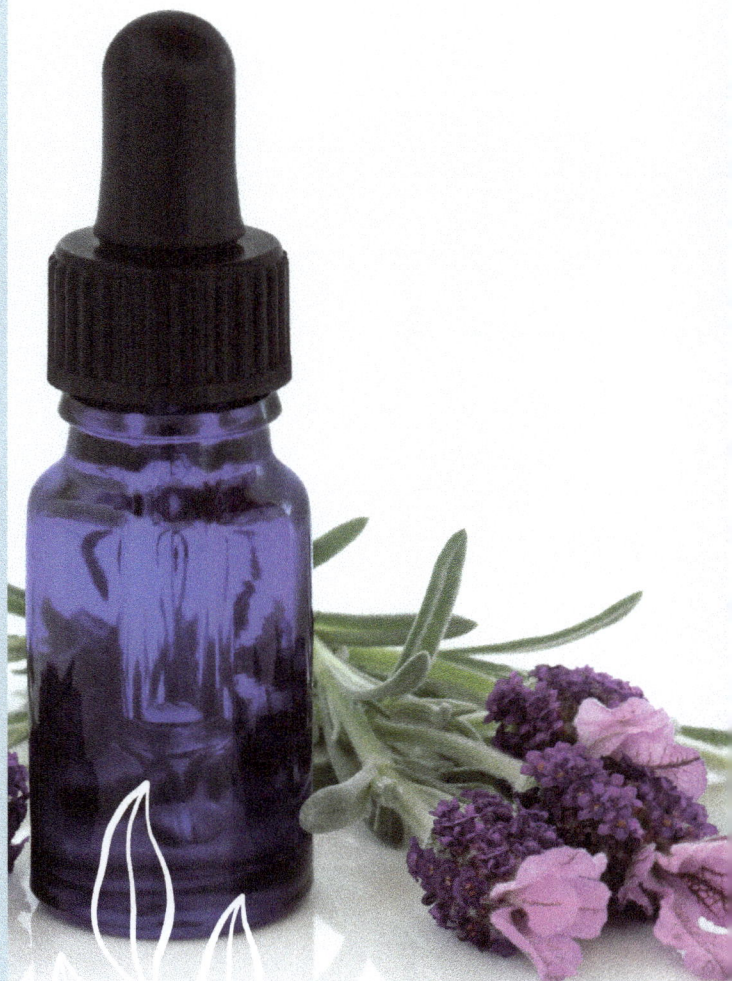

RESOURCES

This chapter will provide a few resources that can help you be successful as an aromatherapy teacher. These resources can also help you in creating your materials to hand out during class.

In this Chapter:

1. Forms for scheduling a one-hour and two-hour workshop or class. Become acquainted with all of the resources here and use them as needed.
2. Class outline for developing your first class.

WORKSHEET: ONE-HOUR WORKSHOP

	Duration	Subject	Activity/ Materials
10:00 AM			
10:10 AM			
10:20 AM			
10:30 AM			
10:40 AM			
10:50 AM			
11:00 AM			
After–Hours Activities			

WORKSHEET:
TWO-HOUR WORKSHOP

	Duration	Subject	Activity/ Materials
10:00 AM			
10:15 AM			
10:30 AM			
10:45 AM			
11:00 AM			
11:15 AM			
11:30 AM			
11:45 AM			
12:00 AM			
After–Hours Activities			

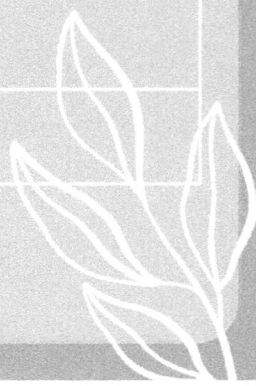

ESSENTIAL OIL CLASS OUTLINE

Use the following outline to help guide you in structuring your class. You can add the crucial pieces into your outline now.

Your Name, Instructor

Theme: _____

Topic: _____

Ice Breaker: _____

INTRODUCTION

1. Attention Material [For ex: PowerPoint slide will be shown]
2. _____
3. _____

(*Transition*) Let's talk about this oil: _____

BODY

1. _____
2. _____
3. _____

(*Transition*) Safety Concerns..._____

1. _____
2. _____
3. _____

(Transition) Look at their benefits..._____

(Transition) Let's summarize.

CONCLUSION

1. Summary _____
2. _____
3. _____
   _____

1. Upcoming Events _____
2. _____
3. _____
   _____

ONE-HOUR CLASS OUTLINE

Lecture (15 minutes): Introduce aromatherapy and the oils you're teaching about.

Questions / Stories (10 minutes): Share YouTube videos, PowerPoint slides, testimonials, or other media that go along with your lecture. This is also a great time to encourage students to ask a few questions about the course material.

Blending Project (20 minutes): Choose a simple recipe—one that doesn't take a lot of time to make. Offer your students different options with choosing their essential oils or have printed recipes for them to follow.

Discussion (10 minutes): Question and answer time. Share about how to use the blend the students made.

Summary (5 minutes): Remind students what they've learned—also use this time to advertise your next class.

TWO-HOUR CLASS OUTLINE

In the two-hour class, you will have time to make two essential oil blends or products.

Ice-Breaker and Introduction (10 minutes): Choose a fun activity to introduce the class to the theme/topic.

Lecture (10 minutes): Depending on your theme, you can discuss the problem and solution (for instance, household store-bought cleaners vs. natural cleaners). This could include video, PowerPoint presentations, and/or show and tell.

Questions / PowerPoint (15 minutes): Share stories about the topic. Take questions from students, etc.

Blending Project (20 minutes): Hands-on activities using the essential oils discussed in the lecture.

Break (15 minutes): Restroom breaks and snacks.

Blending Project (20 minutes): Hands-on activity using the essential oils discussed in the lecture. If you choose not to make a second blend, give 10 minutes to the first blending section and use the other 10 minutes to have students share about their blend.

Break (15 minutes): This is an excellent time to allow students to share their needs and/or look at the book table at items for sale.

Summary and Q&A Session (15 minutes): Remind students of what they've learned and leave them wanting more. Promote products and future events at this time.

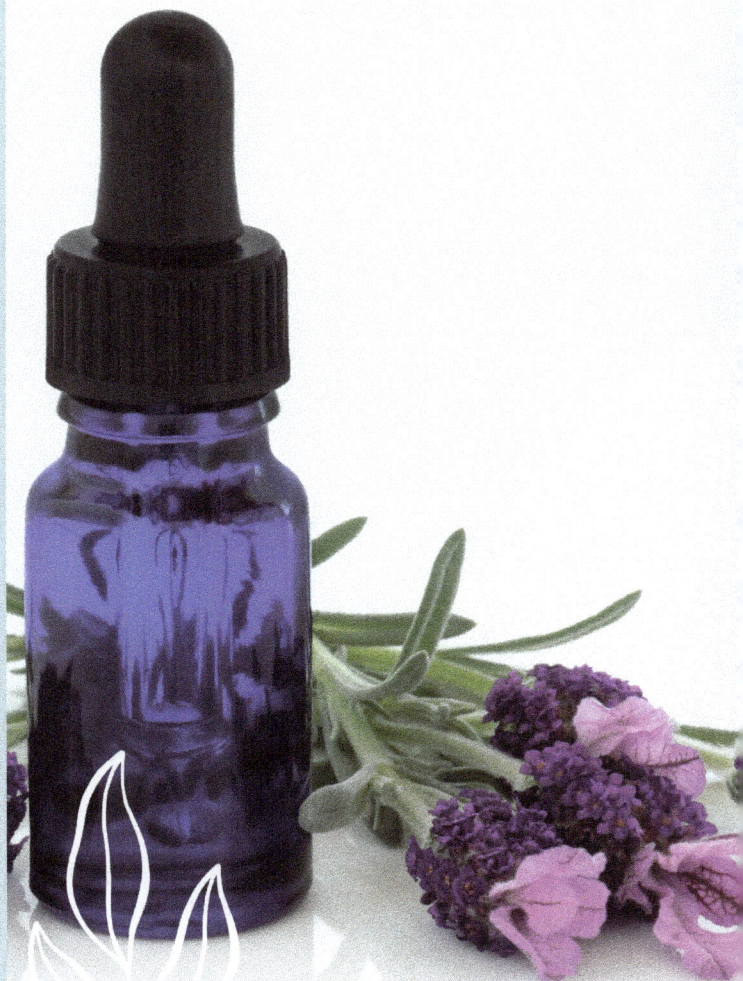

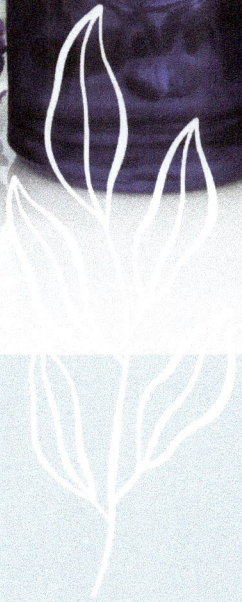

BASIC RECIPES

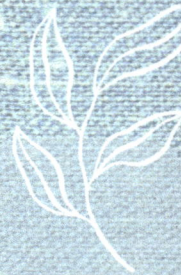

U se these simple recipes as a guideline for creating recipes for your class. You can formulate your essential oil blend that will deliver the healing benefits or fragrance you are seeking.

The recipes below are based on blending by notes, but you can easily use another method such as blending by chemistry or blending by botany simply by changing the formula to match your needs. Of course, there is plenty of room for creativity, as there are no hard and fast rules when it comes to creating your unique blend. Feel free to change these to suit your needs!

MASSAGE OIL BLEND

Here is an easy-to-follow basic recipe for making massage blends! You get to decide which essential oils to use depending on the type of massage and effect you are looking to achieve.

What You Will Need:

- 1 ounce (30 ml) Carrier Oil, Lotion, or Gel
- 9–15 drops Top Note Essential Oil
- 6–10 drops Middle Note Essential Oil
- 3–5 drops Base Note Essential Oil
- Plastic Bottle

What To Do:

1. Pour your carrier oil, lotion, or gel into a clean bottle.
2. Add your essential oils one drop at a time, starting with your base note, followed by the middle note, then the top note.
3. Shake well to mix oils and carrier together.
4. Add a label with the name, ingredients, and date created.
5. Use as normal.

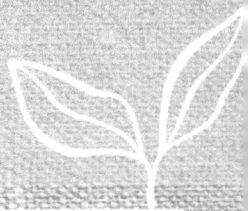

HAND LOTION/OIL BLEND

Here is an easy-to-follow basic recipe for making a hand lotion blend! You can customize this formula with your favorite essential oils and carrier oil.

What You Will Need:

- ½ ounce (30 ml) Almond Oil or Unscented Lotion
- 3 drops Top Note Essential Oil
- 2 drops Middle Note Essential Oil
- 1 drop Base Note Essential Oil
- 15ml Glass Bottle

What To Do:

1. In a glass bottle, add your essential oils, starting with the base, middle, and top notes.
2. Add the Almond oil or another carrier oil and shake to blend oils.
3. After washing hands, massage into hands and wear gloves to retain oil and soften them.

BATH GEL BLEND

Bath blends are easy to create using this basic recipe with a few essential oils!

What You Will Need:

- 1 teaspoon Glycerin, Gel, or Aloe Vera
- 3–12 drops Top Note Essential Oil
- 2–8 drops Middle Note Essential Oil
- 1–4 drops Base Note Essential Oil
- Small Dish or Bowl

What To Do:

1. In a small dish or bowl, add the glycerin or gel as your fixative.
2. Add your essential oils one drop at a time to the fixative and stir well.
3. Pour your bath blend into a stream of warm running bathwater. Enjoy!

Tip: Always check precautions—especially for essential oils that may cause sensitivity to the skin. Be sure to use a 1% dilution or less with children.

JOINT COMPRESS BLEND RECIPE

This is a simple guide to follow when using essential oils in a compress. You will determine which essential oils to use based on the condition or need.

What You Will Need:

- ½ cup Water
- 12 drops Top Note Essential Oil
- 8 drops Middle Note Essential Oil
- 4 drop Base Note Essential Oil
- Small Bowl

What To Do:

1. In a small bowl, add your essential oils, starting with the base, middle, and top notes. Stir to blend well.

2. Using a moistened hand towel or washcloth, soak a cloth in the essential oil blend, then place over the aching joint to relieve pain.

BODY LOTION BLEND

Do you want to try a good body lotion recipe? Why not make your own today by following these simple instructions.

What You Will Need:

- 4 ounces Unscented Lotion, Carrier Oil, or Hydrosol
- 18 drops Top Note Essential Oil
- 12 drops Middle Note Essential Oil
- 6 drops Base Note Essential Oil
- Plastic Bottle or container

What To Do:

1. Place your carrier oil or lotion in your bottle.
2. Add essential oils starting with your base note essential oil first, followed by the middle note, then the top note essential oil.
3. Recap and shake well to mix.
4. Use as normal.

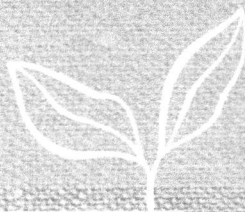

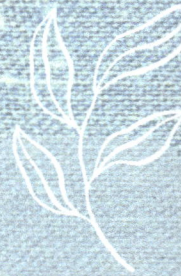

ROOM SPRAY BLEND

Here's an easy room spray recipe you can make in a minute. Using a room spray is a great way to freshen your surroundings and brighten things up! Not only will the essential oils make your space smell great, but you will also be reaping the health benefits of the essential oils as well. The possibilities for this room spray recipe are endless!

What You Will Need:

- 4 ounces Hydrosol, Floral Water or Distilled Water
- 1 tablespoon Glycerin (as a fixative)
- 18–30 drops Top Note Essential Oil
- 12–20 drops Middle Note Essential Oil
- 6–10 drops Base Note Essential Oil
- Glass or Plastic Spray Bottle

What To Do:

1. Add the fixative (Glycerin or Witch Hazel if making a facial spray) in a clean spray bottle.
2. Add your essential oil to the fixative, starting with the base, middle, and top notes. Shake well.
3. Pour the Hydrosol or floral water into the bottle and shake to mix contents well.
4. If you want to make this a facial spray instead, use three ounces of Hydrosol with one ounce of Witch Hazel.

Tip: If using around children or pets, please check precautions for the essential oils you choose.

LINEN SPRAY BLEND

Use this unique blend to help with insomnia or to freshen your bed linens. When using essential oils for your spray, don't forget to determine if they should be stimulating or relaxing!

What You Will Need:

- 8 ounces Hydrosol, Floral Water, or Distilled Water
- 1 tablespoon Glycerin
- 60 drops Top Note Essential Oil
- 40 drops Middle Note Essential Oil
- 20 drops Base Note Essential Oil
- Glass or Plastic Spray Bottle

What To Do:

1. In a clean spray bottle, add the fixative (Glycerin).
2. Add your essential oil to the fixative, starting with the base, middle, and top notes. Shake well.
3. Pour the Hydrosol or floral water into the bottle and shake to mix contents well.
4. Spray on bedspread and linens before making the bed.

BATH SALTS BLEND

For this basic bath salts recipe, you can use Dead Sea, Himalayan, or Epsom salts. This excellent blend will ease achy muscles and soothe away the stress of the day. Your bath salts can be made in advance and stored in a pretty container for convenience.

What You Will Need:

- 2 cups Epsom Salts
- 1 cup Sea Salts
- 1 cup Baking Soda
- 30 drops Top Note Essential Oil
- 20 drops Middle Note Essential Oil
- 10 drops Base Note Essential Oil
- Wide Mouth Jar or container

What To Do:

1. In a container, add your essential oils, starting with the base note, followed by the middle note, then finally the top note. Stir to mix well.
2. Add sea salts and mix well to saturate the salts with the oils thoroughly.
3. In a running bath, add bath salts and swish around in the tub to mix thoroughly.

Tip: Be sure to check precautions for oils that may cause skin sensitivity. Not recommended for children.

SALT SCRUB BLEND

Salt scrubs are great for sloughing off dead skin cells and increasing circulation. For this basic salt scrub recipe, you can choose which salt you prefer, such as Dead Sea, Himalayan, or Epsom salts. Try it for painful joints and achy muscles as well. Your salt scrub can be made fresh each time, or you may want to make some up and store in a pretty container for when the time is right.

What You Will Need:

- ½ cup Sea Salts
- 2–4 ounces Carrier Oil (your choice)
- 9–12 drops Top Note Essential Oil
- 6–8 drops Middle Note Essential Oil
- 3–4 drops Base Note Essential Oil
- Wide Mouth Jar or container

What To Do:

1. In a container, add your carrier oil, such as Almond or Coconut oil. Add your essential oils starting with the base note, followed by the middle note, then finally the top note. Stir to mix well.
2. Add sea salts and mix well to saturate the salts with the oils thoroughly.
3. In the shower or bath, scrub the salt solution into the skin in upward motions toward the heart and in the direction of the lymph flow.

Tip: Be sure to check precautions for oils that may cause skin sensitivity. Not recommended for children.

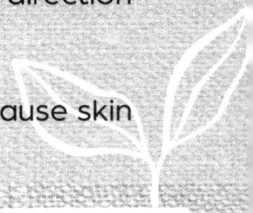

HAIR OIL BLEND

Making your hair shinier and healthier is now possible without spending a fortune on name-brand products. Essential oils can penetrate deeply into your scalp, nourishing the hair follicle, stimulating growth while at the same time inhibiting hair loss. Try this recipe for treating eczema, psoriasis, or stimulating growth!

What You Will Need:

- 1 cup Almond Oil
- 30 drops Top Note Essential Oil
- 20 drops Middle Note Essential Oil
- 10 drops Base Note Essential Oil
- Plastic or Glass Bottle

What To Do:

1. Add your essential oils in a plastic or glass bottle, starting with the base, middle, and top notes. Mix well.
2. Add the Almond oil or another carrier oil to the bottle, replace the lid and shake to blend.
3. To use, massage hair oil into the scalp and let sit for 10–15 minutes. Wash hair as usual.

HAIR SHAMPOO BLEND

Here's an easy way to enhance your shampoo with a delightful formula of essential oils perfect for you! You may even want to purchase a few more ingredients and make your shampoo, avoiding all of those fillers and unnecessary chemicals store-bought shampoos contain, leaving your hair and skin super soft and silky smooth.

What You Will Need:

- 250 ml Shampoo
- 30 drops Top Note Essential Oil
- 20 drops Middle Note Essential Oil
- 10 drops Base Note Essential Oil
- Plastic or Glass Bottle

What To Do:

1. In a plastic bottle or using your existing shampoo bottle, add your essential oils starting with the base note, followed by the middle note, then the top note. Mix well.
2. To use, massage hair shampoo into the scalp and wash hair as usual.

SALVE OINTMENT BLEND

Ointments and salves are good to have on hand when first-aid care is needed. Choose essential oils that can provide antibacterial or antiseptic healing benefits for cuts and wounds.

What You Will Need:

- ½–1 cup Olive Oil or another Carrier Oil
- 2 teaspoons Beeswax
- 9 drops Top Note Essential Oil
- 6 drops Middle Note Essential Oil
- 3 drops Base Note Essential Oil
- Small Jar or Tin

What To Do:

1. Using a double glass boiler, heat the oil over hot water. If you prefer, you can heat oil in a pan directly over the burner on low heat or in a microwave until warm.
2. Add the beeswax and stir until melted.
3. Let the oil cool slightly (not too long, or it will set up).
4. Add the essential oils, starting with the base, middle, and top notes. Stir to blend.
5. Pour mixture into jars or tins immediately. If the mixture begins to set, reheat slightly.

Tip: For variation, you can use solid Coconut oil and omit the beeswax. You may also want to add 6–8 Vitamin E oil capsules as a preservative.

SMELLING SALTS BLEND

When sinuses are congested, making it impossible to breathe, try using these scented salts!

What You Will Need:

- 1 cup Epsom Salts
- 1 cup Sea Salts
- 30 drops Top Note Essential Oil
- 20 drops Middle Note Essential Oil
- 10 drops Base Note Essential Oil
- Jar with Lid
- Bowl

What To Do:

1. In a bowl, add your essential oils, starting with the base note, the middle note, and the top note. Mix well.
2. In a jar, add your salts. Add the essential oil blend and stir to blend thoroughly. Replace lid.
3. When needed, open the jar and take a deep whiff to open sinuses.

BATH TEA BLEND

For an extraordinary bathing experience, try adding dried herbs, flower petals, and oils to your running bath for a relaxing time!

What You Will Need:

- 2 cups Herbs (Lavender flowers, Mint leaves, etc.)
- 1 cup Sea Salts (your choice)
- 6 drops Top Note Essential Oil
- 4 drops Middle Note Essential Oil
- 2 drops Base Note Essential Oil

What To Do:

1. In a mixing bowl, add dried herbs and flower petals to sea salts and stir to blend.
2. Add essential oils starting with the base oil, the middle note, and the top note. Stir to mix well.
3. Store in an airtight container jar. Add a scoopful of the mixture into a cotton or linen bag and hang under running bathwater. If you do not have a bag, add the mixture directly into the bath. Enjoy!

PERFUME OIL BLEND

Whether soft and subtle or exotic and romantic, you can easily make any fragrance you desire. This basic recipe can be changed and adapted to your signature style, depending on what you like. Keep track of what you add or change, so you'll know how to make your favorite blends at a later time.

What You Will Need:

- ½ ounce Jojoba Oil
- 9 drops Top Note Essential Oil
- 6 drops Middle Note Essential Oil
- 3 drops Base Note Essential Oil
- Dark Bottle

What To Do:

1. Add your carrier oil, such as Jojoba, to a clean, dark glass bottle.
2. When adding essential oils, start with the base note, then add the middle note, followed by the top note. As you add each one, check the scent to ensure it is what you are looking for.
3. Allow your blend to sit for 48 hours up to six weeks. The longer it sits, the stronger the fragrance will intensify.
4. Remove the cap and see if it has the desired scent you are looking for. If not, you can add more essential oils and let it sit longer until you get the desired scent.
5. At the end of this maturing process, your perfume should be ready. Store your perfume in a dark, cool place. Don't forget to name your creation!

Tip: You will have to play around with scents for a little bit before hitting on what you like. Make sure that you write each ratio of every essential oil used in a particular scent, as nothing can be more frustrating than actually coming up with the fragrance of your dreams and then not remembering how you ended up making it.

BATH OIL BLEND

After a long day, soaking in a warm bath with a relaxing essential oil blend can be a sensual treat. Not only does it help take the edge off tense muscles, but it also ensures a better night's sleep. For early risers, starting your day with a refreshing essential oil blend at bath time may be more your speed, kick-starting your morning! Of course, a bath essential oil blend for achy joints can be helpful any time of day!

What You Will Need:

- 1 cup Almond Oil or Coconut Oil
- 30 drops Top Note Essential Oil
- 20 drops Middle Note Essential Oil
- 10 drops Base Note Essential Oil
- Corked container
- Crystal beads, dried flowers, tiny seashells, etc. (optional)

What To Do:

1. Pour the carrier oil through a funnel into the corked container, leaving about an inch at the top.
2. Start with the base note when adding essential oils, then add the middle note, followed by the top note. As you add each one, check the scent to ensure it is what you are looking for.
3. Cork the container and agitate the bottle gently.
4. Let it sit for 2-3 days before using. Add decor to your bottle.
5. For use, pour ½ - 1 teaspoon into the palm of your hand and gently massage into your body after a bath.

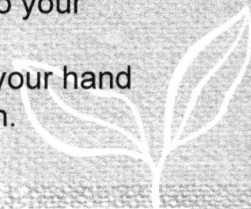

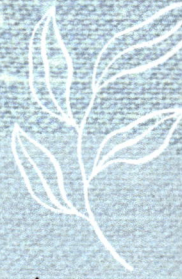

FACIAL OIL BLEND

Formulate a blend that will heal and nourish your complexion to treat those special skin conditions such as extra dry or mature skin. Be sure to match your skin type for the best results.

What You Will Need:

- 1 ounce Almond Oil or Another Carrier Oil
- 9 drops Top Note Essential Oil
- 6 drops Middle Note Essential Oil
- 3 drops Base Note Essential Oil
- Small Bottle

What To Do:

1. In a small bottle, add essential oils starting with the base oil, followed by the middle note, then finally the top note.
2. Add the Almond oil or another carrier oil to your blend and shake to mix.
3. After thoroughly washing your face, apply several drops of your blend to trouble areas and gently massage into your face using upward strokes. Leave on overnight.

NASAL INHALER BLEND

Filling a blank nasal inhaler with your favorite essential oil blend is an effective way to experience the therapeutic power of essential oils when suffering from respiratory issues or emotional issues. Inhalers are great to use for colds, flu, headaches, allergies, and lung and chest congestion. These are small enough to carry in a pocket or purse and have on hand for immediate relief. Add 15–18 drops of your essential oil blend to your inhaler.

What You Will Need:

- 9 drops Top Note Essential Oil
- 6 drops Middle Note Essential Oil
- 3 drops Base Note Essential Oil
- Glass or Plastic Disposable Dropper
- Small Plastic Inhaler

What To Do:

1. In a small bottle, add essential oils starting with the base oil, followed by the middle note, then finally the top note. Stir to mix well.
2. Use a glass or disposal dropper to fill the nasal inhaler.
3. Carry and take a whiff as needed.

FOOT SCRUB BLEND

Aromatic foot scrubs are a great way to get rid of rough, cal-loused skin on your heels, leaving them smooth and silky for sandals and summertime fun!

What You Will Need:

- ¼ cup Ground Oatmeal
- ¼ cup Cornmeal
- 1 tablespoon Sea Salt
- 1 teaspoon Moisturizer or Lotion
- 6 drops Top Note Essential Oil
- 4 drops Middle Note Essential Oil
- 2 drops Base Note Essential Oil
- Spring Water

What To Do:

1. In a small bowl, combine all of the dry ingredients.
2. Add enough water to form a gritty paste.
3. Add essential oils starting with the base oil, the middle note, and the top note. Stir to mix well.
4. Massage into feet after a shower or bath, scrubbing all the rough areas. Rinse and dry.
5. Squeeze a teaspoon of moisturizer into your palm, then add a few drops of your favorite essential oil like pep-permint, eucalyptus, or rosemary and stir with your fin-ger. Massage into feet and legs in an upward motion.

FOOT POWDER BLEND

For sweaty feet, try using a foot powder with tea tree essential oil or rosemary essential oil that acts as a natural deodorizer and helps with excess perspiration. Essential oils with antifungal properties aid in preventing athlete's foot and other fungus issues.

What You Will Need:

- 2 ½ tablespoons Arrowroot Powder
- 3 drops Top Note Essential Oil
- 2 drops Middle Note Essential Oil
- 1 drop Base Note Essential Oil
- 1 teaspoon Moisturizer or Lotion
- Spring Water

What To Do:

1. In a small bowl, add the Arrowroot powder.
2. Add essential oils starting with the base oil, the middle note, and the top note. Stir to mix well.
3. Dust feet with powder before putting on socks and shoes.

FOOT OIL BLEND

Sometimes your feet just need some tender loving care! Try this oil after shopping, hiking, or exploring all day, and your feet are worn out! You can be creative and try different carrier oils and essential oils that work best for you.

What You Will Need:

- 1 tablespoon Almond Oil
- 1 tablespoon Olive Oil
- 1 tablespoon Wheatgerm Oil
- 6 drops Top Note Essential Oil
- 4 drops Middle Note Essential Oil
- 2 drops Base Note Essential Oil
- Small Bottle

What To Do:

1. In a small bottle, add the carrier oils.
2. Add essential oils starting with the base oil, the middle note, and the top note. Shake to blend.
3. Massage into feet and heels after a long day.

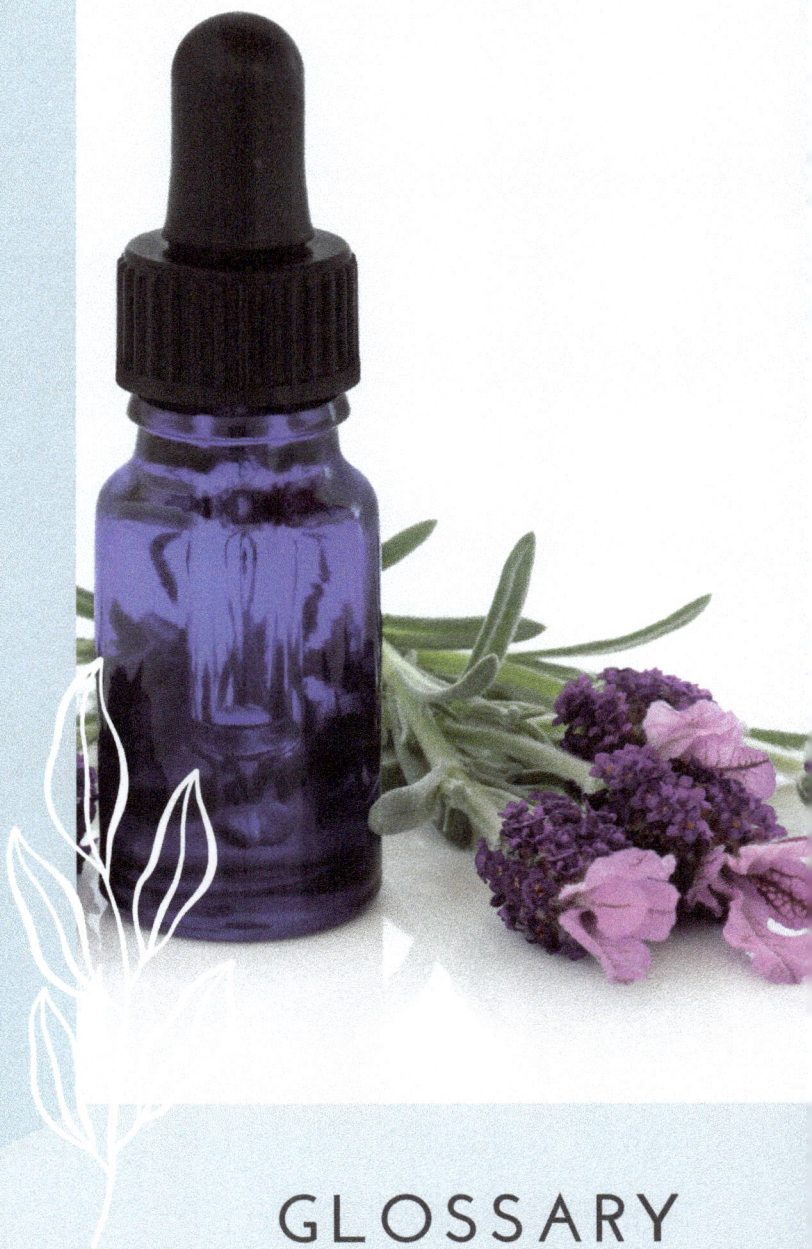

GLOSSARY OF ESSENTIAL OIL TERMS

Abortifacient	A substance or agent that can induce an abortion.
Absorption Rate	The rate at which an essential oil or carrier oil penetrates the skin over a given period of time (can be subjective).
Absolute	A concentrated, highly aromatic, oily mixture extracted from plants produces a waxy mass called concrete through solvent extraction techniques. The lower molecular weight, fragrant compounds are extracted from the concrete into ethanol. When the ethanol evaporates, the absolute is left behind.
Adulterate	To make impure by adding extraneous, improper, or inferior ingredients.
Alcohol	The word used by itself usually refers to Ethyl Alcohol or Ethanol, the primary solvent used to carry perfume for extracts, colognes. When referring to its chemical name, it refers to the chemical group R–OH.
Aldehyde	The chemical group R–CHO. The word by itself usually refers to shorter (C6–C12) straight–chain (aliphatic) aldehydes used in perfumery.
Analgesic	An agent that relieves pain by acting upon the peripheral and central nervous systems.
Anaphrodisiac	The decline or absence of sexual desire.
Anosmic	Having no sense of smell.
Anthelmintic	An agent that destroys or causes the expulsion of parasitic intestinal worms.
Anti–allergenic	A substance capable of preventing an allergic reaction.

Anti-anxiety	An agent capable of preventing or reducing anxiety.
Anti-arthritic	An agent that alleviates arthritis by providing therapy to relieve the symptoms of joint inflammation.
Anti-asthmatic	An agent that provides relief from asthma or halts an asthmatic attack.
Antibacterial	An agent capable of destroying or inhibiting the growth or reproduction of bacteria.
Antibiotic	A substance used to stop a bacterial infection from spreading and prevents the growth of bacteria in the body.
Anticatarrhal	A substance effective against catarrh or inflammation of the mucous membranes, especially of the nose and throat.
Anti-coagulant	A substance that inhibits the clotting of blood by blocking the action of clotting factors or platelets.
Anti-convulsant	An agent that helps prevent or reduce the severity of epileptic or other convulsive seizures.
Antidepressant	A substance or an agent used to alleviate mood disorders such as depression and anxiety and prevent clinical depression.
Antidontalgic	A substance that can relieve a toothache.
Anti-emetic	An agent that prevents or alleviates nausea and vomiting.

Antifungal	A substance used to treat fungal infections such as athlete's foot, ringworm, candidiasis (thrush), and serious conditions such as cryptococcal meningitis.
Anti-galactagogue	An agent that inhibits or lessens the secretion and flow of milk.
Antihistamine	A compound that inhibits the production of histamine, primarily used in the treatment of allergies and colds.
Anti-hemorrhagic	A substance that prevents or stops bleeding.
Anti-infectious	An agent capable of stopping the colonization of a microscopic organism such as a virus or bacteria.
Anti-inflammatory	A substance that prevents or reduces certain types of inflammation such as swelling, tenderness, fever, and pain.
Antimicrobial	An agent capable of destroying or inhibiting the growth of microorganisms.
Antineuralgic	An agent that relieves neuralgia, intense burning or stabbing pain caused by irritation of or damage to a nerve caused by disease, inflammation, or infection.
Antioxidant	A substance that retards or inhibits oxidation.
Anti-parasitic	An agent that destroys and inhibits the growth of parasites.
Anti-phlogistic	A substance that relieves inflammation and fever.
Anti-pruritic	An agent that prevents or relieves itching.

Anti-putrescent	A substance that inhibits or counteracts a putrefaction odor such as decay, foul smell, rot, and decomposition.
Anti-pyretic	An agent that reduces a fever.
Anti-rheumatic	An agent that suppresses the manifestation of rheumatic disease and can delay the progression of the disease process in inflammatory arthritis; it relieves the symptoms of any painful or immobilizing disorder of the musculoskeletal system.
Anti-sclerotic	An agent that helps to prevent the hardening of arteries or is affected with sclerosis.
Anti-scorbutic	Refers to an agent that cures or prevents scurvy.
Antiseptic	Refers to a substance capable of preventing infection by inhibiting the growth and reproduction of microorganisms.
Antispasmodic	An agent that relieves or prevents spasms, particularly of smooth muscle.
Anti-sudorific	A substance that is capable of inhibiting the secretion of sweat.
Anti-toxic	An agent that neutralizes the action of a toxin or poison.
Anti-tussive	A substance that suppresses the body's urge to cough.
Anti-venomous	An anti-toxin active against the venom of a snake, spider, or other venomous animal or insect.

Antiviral	An agent or substance capable of destroying a virus and inhibits it from spreading and reproducing.
Aperitif	A substance taken to stimulate the appetite before a meal.
Aphrodisiac	A substance that arouses or intensifies sexual desire and function.
Aromachology	The science, coined by the Olfactory Research Fund, is dedicated to studying the interrelationship between psychology and aroma.
Aromatherapy	The art and science of using essential oils to heal common ailments and complaints. Therapy with aroma can be beneficial for stress or emotionally trigger problems such as insomnia and headaches. The term "aromatherapy" was coined by a French chemist, R.M. Gattefosse.
Aromatic	Refers to the Benzene ring structure found in many organic compounds. However, the term in perfumery refers to the rich aroma displayed by Balsamic notes.
Astringent	A substance that draws together or constricts body tissues and effectively stops the flow of blood or other secretions.
Attar (Otto)	From the ancient Persian word "to smell sweet." Attar or Otto refers to essential oil obtained by distillation and, in particular, the Bulgarian Rose, an extremely precious perfumery material.
Bactericide	A substance that kills bacteria.

Balsamic	A soothing substance having the qualities of balsam.
Bechic	An agent that relieves coughing.
Botanical Name	A scientific name in Latin that conforms to the International Code of Botanical Nomenclature (ICBN) is of a specific plant species that clearly distinguishes it from other plants that share the same common name. The purpose of a formal name is to have a single name that is accepted and used worldwide for a particular plant or plant group.
Calming	A substance that causes a sense of serenity, tranquility, and peace.
Calmative	An agent that has relaxing or sedating properties.
Carminative	An agent that induces the expulsion of gas from the stomach or intestines; settles the digestive system and relieves flatulence.
Carrier Oil	A vegetable fatty oil used to dilute essential oils for application to the skin or massage.
Chemotypes	The same botanical species occurring in other forms due to different growth conditions.
Cholagogue	An agent which promotes the discharge of bile from the system, purging it downward.
Cicatrisant	An agent that promotes the formation of scar tissue.
Circulatory Stimulant	A substance that temporarily increases circulation and invigorates the circulatory system.

CO2 Extracts	Oils extracted by the carbon dioxide method are commonly referred to as CO2 Extracts or CO2s for short. Essential oils processed by this method are considered superior. None of the constituents have been harmed by heat, have a closer aroma to the natural source, and generally thicker oils.
Cold-Pressed	Refers to a method of extraction where no external heat is applied during the process.
Common Name	The familiar name used for a plant. Names such as chamomile, lavender, orange, or eucalyptus may refer to more than one species yet go by the same name. It is necessary to know its botanical name for clarity.
Concrete	A waxy concentrated semi-solid essential oil extract is made from plant material used to make an absolute.
Cooling	A substance that offers relief from heat and has a calming effect.
Cordial	A cordial is an invigorating and stimulating preparation that is intended for a medicinal purpose. Cordials were traditionally a weak alcoholic beverage flavored with essential oils, fruit essences, or plant extracts and sweetened.
Cytophylactic	An agent that increases the leukocyte activity in its ability to defend the body against infection.
Decoction	A herbal preparation made by boiling the plant material and reducing it into a concentration.

Decongestant	An agent that treats sinus congestion by reducing swelling.
Demulcent	An agent that soothes irritated mucous membranes and relieves pain and inflammation.
Deodorant	A substance that removes or conceals body odors.
Depurative	A substance that is purgative or used for purifying.
Dermatitis	Inflammation of the skin.
Detoxifier	A substance that helps to detoxify and remove impurities from the blood and body.
Diaphoretic	An agent that promotes perspiration.
Diffuser	A device used to disperse the aromatic molecules of essential oils into the air.
Digestive Support	A substance or formula that helps to improve the digestive system.
Disinfectant	A substance or agent that destroys neutralizes, or inhibits the growth of disease-carrying microorganisms.
Distillation	A method of extraction used in the manufacture of essential oils.
Diuretic	A substance that increases the flow of urine, thus removing water from the body.
Dram	A unit of measurement equaling 1/8 of an ounce.
Emmenagogue	A substance used to stimulate blood flow in the pelvic area and uterus; some stimulate menstruation.

Emollient	A substance that softens and soothes the skin.
Endocrine	The secretion of an endocrine ductless gland, a hormone.
Essential Oil	An aromatic, volatile liquid consisting of odorous principles from plant extracts.
Exocrine	That which pertains to a gland with a duct secreting directly onto the outside surface of an organism.
Expectorant	An agent that promotes the secretion or expulsion of phlegm, mucus, or other matter from the respiratory passages.
Expression	An extraction method where plant materials are pressed to obtain the essential oil.
Exudates	A natural substance secreted by plants that can be spontaneous or result from damage to the plant.
Febrifuge	An agent that reduces fever.
Fixative	A natural or synthetic substance used to slow down the evaporation of volatile components in perfume and improve stability when added to more volatile components.
Fixed Oils	Vegetable oils are obtained from plants that are fatty and non-volatile.
Fractionated Oil	A process in which oils are re-distilled, either to have terpenes or other substances removed.
Fungicidal	A substance that destroys or inhibits the growth of fungi.

Galactagogue	An agent that induces milk secretion.
Hydro Diffusion	A method of extracting essential oils in which steam at atmospheric pressure is passed through the plant material from the top of the extraction chamber, resulting in oils that retain the plant's original aroma and are less harsh than steam distillation.
Hydrosol (Floral Water)	The water resulting from the distillation of essential oils, which still contains some of the properties of the plant material from the extraction process.
Hypertension	Arterial disease in which chronic high blood pressure is the primary symptom.
Hypertensive	An agent that raises blood pressure.
Hypotension	Abnormally low blood pressure.
Immunostimulant	An agent that stimulates an immune response.
Immune Support	An agent that supports the immune system and assists in the resistance to infection by a specific pathogen.
Infused Oil	Oil produced by steeping the macerated botanical material in the liquid until it has taken on some of the plant material's properties.
Infusion	The process of making a herbal remedy by steeping plant material in water to extract its soluble principles.
Insecticide	A substance that repels and kills insects.

Massage Therapy	The manipulation of the body's soft tissue to enhance health and is known to affect the circulation of blood and the flow of blood and lymph, reduce muscular tension or flaccidity, affect the nervous system through stimulation or sedation, and enhance tissue healing.
Mucolytic	Denotes an enzyme that breaks down mucus.
Nervine	An agent that has a soothing or calming effect upon the nerves.
Neurotoxin	A substance that is poisonous or destructive to nerve tissue.
Oleoresin	Natural resinous exudation from plants or aromatic liquid extracted from botanical material.
Olfaction	Refers to the sense of smell.
Olfactory Bulb	The bulblike distal end of the olfactory lobe center is where the smell is processed and passed onto other areas of the brain.
Orifice Reducer	A small plastic insert inside the glass bottle that acts as a dropper. To use, tip the bottle to count out the number of drops.
Oxidation	The process in which the addition of oxygen to an organic molecule, or the removal of electrons or hydrogen from the molecule.
Pathogenic	An agent that causes disease.

Phytohormones	Plant substances mimicking the actions of human hormones. Plant hormones in the plant control or regulate germination, growth, metabolism, or other physiological activities.
Phytotherapy	The use of natural plant extracts for medicinal purposes as in the treatment of disease.
Pipette	This is a plastic dropper used to dispense essential oil from a bottle into another bottle or container.
Pomade	Perfumed fat obtained during the effleurage extraction method.
Prophylactic	An act of preventing disease or infection.
Rectification	A process of re–distilling essential oils to remove certain constituents and purify it.
Resin	A natural substance exuded from trees; prepared resins are oleoresins from which the essential oil has been removed.
Rubefacient	A substance that irritates the skin, causing redness.
Sedative	An agent with a soothing, calming, or tranquilizing effect on the body that relieves anxiety, stress, irritability, or excitement.
Shelf Life	The amount of time a carrier or base oil will remain fresh before oxidizing and become rancid.
Stimulant	A substance that raises the physiological levels of the central nervous system.

Stomachic	A substance that aids in digestion in the stomach and improves appetite.
Sudorific	An agent that causes or increases sweat.
Synergy	Several substances or agents working together in harmony to produce a greater effect than the sum of the individual agents. A synergistic blend of essential oils would be one with the correct proportions of oils with a greater impact than an individual oil.
Terpene	One of a class of hydrocarbons with an empiric formula of C10H16, occurring in essential oils and resins.
Tonic	A substance that gives a feeling of vigor or well-being.
Unguent	A soothing or healing salve, balm, or ointment.
Vasoconstrictor	A substance that causes the vasoconstriction of blood vessels typically increases blood pressure and pupil dilation; vasodilatation is the opposite. It relaxes the smooth muscle walls and causes the opening of blood vessels, lowering blood pressure.
Vein Tonic	A substance that improves and strengthens the functioning of blood vessels.
Vermifuge	An anathematic that expels parasitic worms from the body by either stunning or killing them.
Viscosity	The degree to which a fluid moves and flows under an applied force. With carrier oils, it may be noted as "thin," or "thick," etc.

Volatile	A substance that is unstable and evaporates quickly, such as an essential oil.
Vulnerary	A remedy used in healing or treating wounds and helps to prevent tissue degeneration.
Warming	A substance that raises the temperature slightly.
Wound Healing	An agent that can assist in healing an injury, especially one in which the skin or another external surface that has been torn, pierced, cut, or otherwise broken.

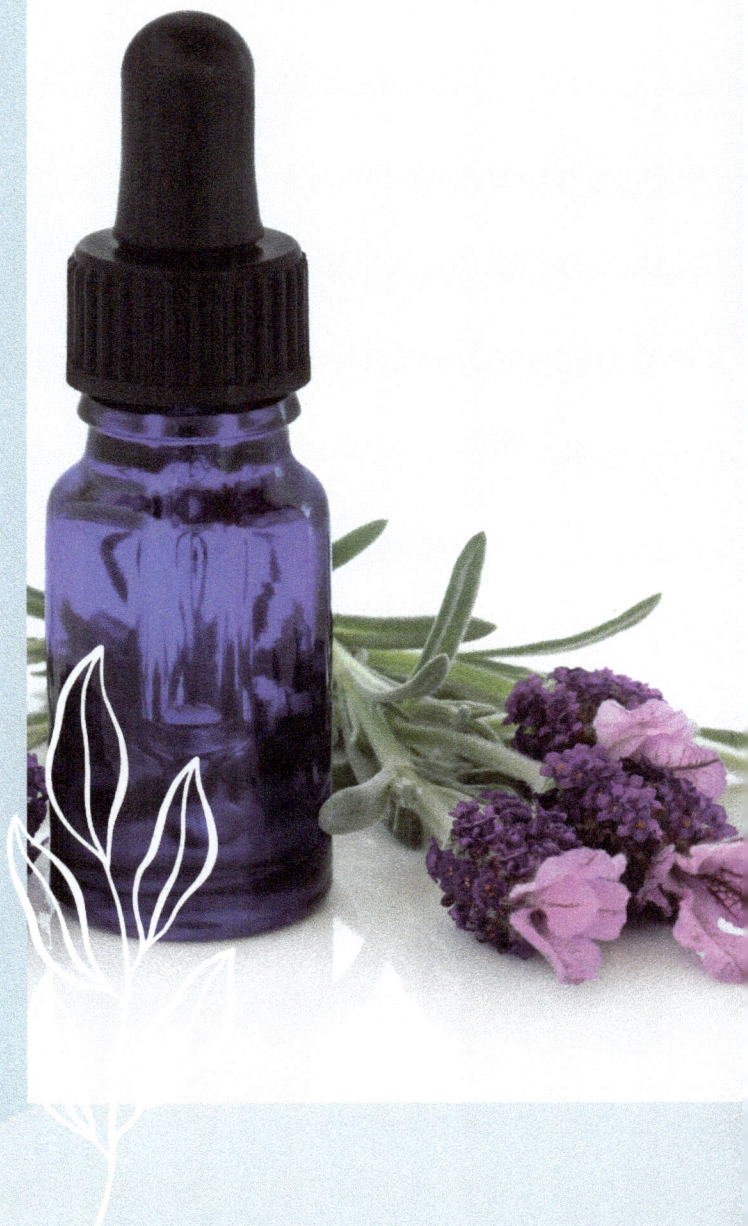

OTHER BOOKS
BY REBECCA PARK TOTILO

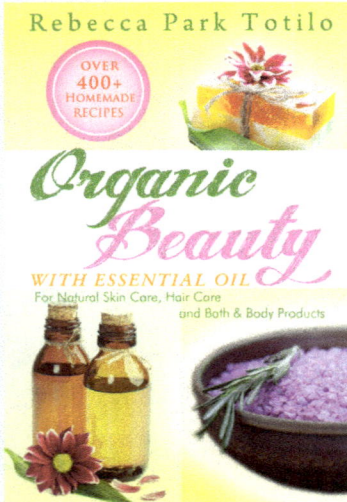

Organic Beauty With Essential Oil: Over 400+ Homemade Recipes for Natural Skin Care, Hair Care and Bath & Body Products

Sweep aside all those harmful chemically-based cosmetics and make your own organic bath and body products at home with the magic of potent essential oils! In this book, you'll find a luxurious array of over 400 Eco-friendly recipes that call for breathtaking fragrances and soothing, rich organic ingredients satisfying you head to toe. Included you'll find helpful can have the confidence knowing which essential oil to use and how much when creating your own body scrub, lip butter, or lotion bar! Discover how easy it is to make bath treats like fragrant shower gels, dreamy bubble baths, luscious creams and lotions, deep cleansing masks and facials for literally pennies using essential oils and ingredients from your kitchen.

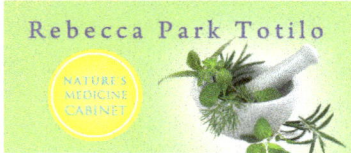

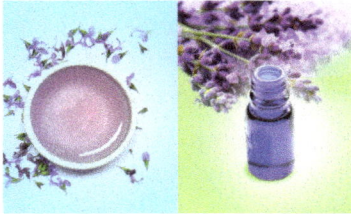

Heal With Essential Oil: Nature's Medicine Cabinet

Using essential oils drawn from nature's own medicine cabinet of flowers, trees, seeds and roots, man can tap into God's healing power to heal oneself from almost any pain. Find relief from many conditions and rejuvenate the body. With over 125 recipes, this practical guide will walk you through in the most easy-to-understand form how to treat common ailments with your essential oils for everyday living. Filled with practical advice on therapeutic blending of oils and safety, a directory of the most effective oils for common ailments and easy to follow remedies chart, and prescriptive blends for aches, pains and sicknesses.

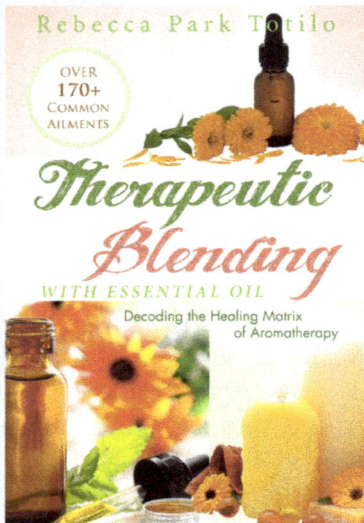

Therapeutic Blending With Essential Oil: Decoding the Healing Matrix of Aromatherapy

Therapeutic Blending With Essential Oil unlocks the healing power of essential oils and guides you through the intricate matrix of aromatherapy, with a compilation of over 170 common ailments. Discover how to properly formulate a blend for any physical or emotional symptom with easy to follow customizable recipes. Now, you can make your own massage oils, hand and body lotions, bath gels, compresses, salve ointments, smelling salts, nasal inhalers and more. This exhaustive guide takes all the guesswork out of blending oils from how many drops to include in a blend, to measuring thick oils, to how often to apply it for acute or chronic conditions. It also shows you how to create a single blend for multiple conditions. Even if you run out of oil for a favorite recipe, this book shows you how to substitute it with another oil.

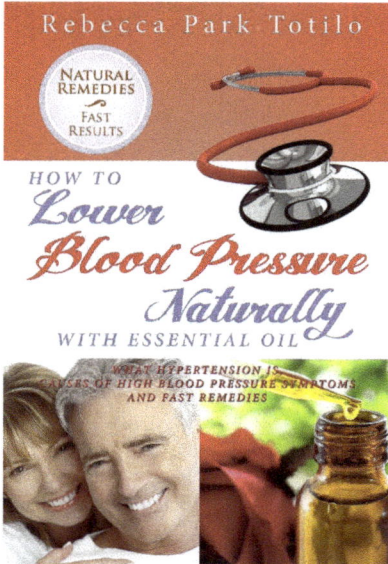

How To Lower Blood Pressure Naturally With Essential Oil: What Hypertension Is, Causes of High Pressure Symptoms and Fast Remedies

One out of three adults have it, and another one-third don't realize it. Oftentimes, it goes undetected for years. Even those who take multiple medications for it still don't have it under control. It's no secret -- high blood pressure is rampant in America. High blood pressure, or hypertension, has become a household term. Between balancing meds and monitoring diets though, are the true causes -- and best treatments -- hidden in the shadows? In How to Lower Blood Pressure Naturally With Essential Oil, Rebecca Park Totilo sheds light on what high blood pressure is, the causes and symptoms of high blood pressure, and which essential oils regulate blood pressure and how to use essential oils as a natural, alternative method.

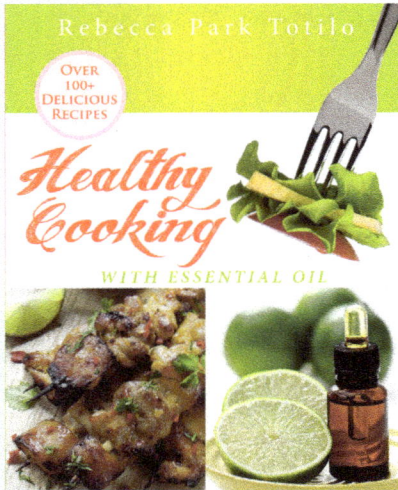

Healthy Cooking with Essential Oil

Imagine transforming an everyday dish into something extraordinary using only a drop or two of essential oil can enliven everything from soups, salads, to main dishes and desserts. Boasting flavor and fragrance, these intense essences can turn a dull, boring meal into something appetizing and delicious. Essential oils are fun, easy-to use and beneficial, compared to the traditional stale, dried herbs and spices found in most pantries today. Healthy food should never be thought of as mere fuel for the body, it should be enjoyed as a multi-sensory experience that brings therapeutic value as well as nourishment. For years we have limited the use of essential oils to scented candles and soaps, in the belief that they were unsafe to consume (and some are!). However, more people are realizing the value of using pure essential oils to enhance their diet. In Healthy Cooking With Essential Oil, you will learn how cooking with essential oils can open up a wealth of creative opportunities in the kitchen.

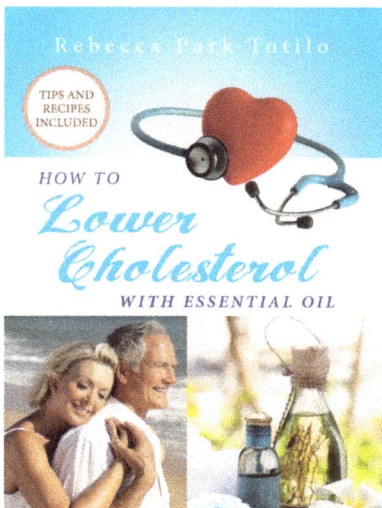

How to Lower Cholesterol with Essential Oil

Take healthy steps now to control high cholesterol and its risk factors with essential oils. People with high cholesterol have twice the risk for heart disease according to the Center for Disease Control and Prevention. What's worse, most folks aren't even aware that they have atherosclerosis until they have a heart attack or stroke. Lowering your cholesterol and triglycerides with essential oils may slow, reduce, or even stop the buildup of dangerous plaque in your arteries causing blockage of blood flow which could result in a heart attack or stroke. In this indispensable guide, author Rebecca Park Totilo presents scientific research supporting the efficacy of certain essential oils for lowering cholesterol, an extensive essential oil and carrier oil directory, natural treatments with recipes, along with easy-to-follow methods of use via inhalation, topically, and ingestion.

www.ingramcontent.com/pod-product-compliance
Lightning Source LLC
Chambersburg PA
CBHW040135270326
41927CB00019B/3394